Telephone Assessment in Primary Care

Telephone Assessment in Primary Care

a practical guide to effective consultation and triage

Sally-Anne Pygall

Founder, Telelearning Ltd, Durham
(www.telelearning.co.uk)

Scion

© **Scion Publishing Ltd, 2023**

First published 2023

ISBN 9781914961366

A CIP catalogue record for this book is available from the British Library.

Scion Publishing Limited
The Old Hayloft, Vantage Business Park, Bloxham Road, Banbury OX16 9UX, UK
www.scionpublishing.com

Important Note from the Publisher
The information contained within this book was obtained by Scion Publishing Ltd from sources believed by us to be reliable. However, while every effort has been made to ensure its accuracy, no responsibility for loss or injury whatsoever occasioned to any person acting or refraining from action as a result of information contained herein can be accepted by the authors or publishers.

Readers are reminded that medicine is a constantly evolving science and while the authors and publishers have ensured that all dosages, applications and practices are based on current indications, there may be specific practices which differ between communities. You should always follow the guidelines laid down by the manufacturers of specific products and the relevant authorities in the country in which you are practising.

Although every effort has been made to ensure that all owners of copyright material have been acknowledged in this publication, we would be pleased to acknowledge in subsequent reprints or editions any omissions brought to our attention.

Registered names, trademarks, etc. used in this book, even when not marked as such, are not to be considered unprotected by law.

Cover design by Andrew Magee Design
Typeset by Evolution Design & Digital Ltd (Kent)
Printed in the UK

Last digit is the print number: 10 9 8 7 6 5 4 3

Contents

Preface

When I was approached about writing a second book on telephone triage and consultation skills, I wasn't sure that I could. I had put so much into my previous book and didn't feel I could do any more. However, I was asked to write it in a different way – a consolidated adaptation to give clinicians a more precise reference book that got to the heart of this difficult and stressful clinical specialty. I also decided to aim it directly at clinicians working only within primary care, whether it be in-hours or out-of-hours.

The pandemic brought telephone care to the heart of every care service and showed what could be achieved using the phone, but it also showed how using the phone to deliver care should be given all due respect and that clinicians need good quality training if they are to do it safely and efficiently. Unfortunately, this isn't always the case and so this book will hopefully go some way to providing the knowledge, tools and techniques that can be used to assess patients over the phone.

I continue to be passionate about telephone care and fervently hope that this book will help you understand how we can help patients without having to see them. Telephone work can be immensely satisfying for the clinician and the patient, but only when it's done well.

Sally-Anne Pygall

About the author

Sally-Anne Pygall is one of the leading experts on telephone triage in the UK, and has an MSc in Evidence Based Practice from the University of York. She runs her own training and consultancy company Telelearning (www.telelearning.co.uk) – a company that specialises in training for clinical and non-clinical staff working in telephone healthcare. As a Senior Nurse with over three decades of experience in this area, Sally-Anne is a fervent advocate of telephone triage. She delivers training on behalf of the Royal College of General Practitioners and has done so for over 10 years, but her main area of training is within general practices and out-of-hours services.

Telephone healthcare carries enormous risks for everyone involved and Sally-Anne understands better than most how many clinicians are ill-prepared for this specialist skill. Her passion for telephone triage and consultations and her aspiration to educate clinicians in carrying out safe and effective triage, are unrivalled. She also trains non-clinical staff in dealing with patients over the phone and works as an Expert Witness across the UK.

Chapter 1
Telephone triage versus telephone consultations

> **Key points**
>
> - Telephone triage and telephone consultations are one and the same thing clinically – an assessment of symptoms over the phone
> - Different terms are usually 'system' requirements, i.e. same-day requests or overflow versus follow-up or patient requests phone call
> - What you call these interactions (triage or consultations) may affect your decision-making
> - Don't prejudge the outcome or the nature of the call
> - Calls that don't involve an assessment of symptoms should be discounted for the learning purposes of this book

1.1 How the telephone is used in primary care

The telephone has been used in primary care since the phone was invented, but the advent of the Covid-19 pandemic in 2020 made many of us change our opinion and practice in how we use the phone.

1.1.1 Pre-pandemic use of the phone

Prior to the pandemic, telephone *triage* was mostly used as a quick method for 'sorting' calls in order of priority for a face-to-face (sometimes shortened to f2f) consultation. This would make sense, as the literal translation of the French word *triage* is 'sorting out'. These triage calls were often used to deal with what could be considered as the 'overflow' once all the day's allocated appointment slots had been used. Any further demand for same-day appointments or 'urgent' cases would be dealt with initially over the phone by the duty doctor. Sometimes the telephone triage list was limited, but in some cases, surgeries would simply add as many calls as was necessary to the 'call-back list', as it is often referred to. This could mean that some lists were mindbogglingly long!

Telephone *consultations* were often allocated more time than a telephone triage and were used either for follow-ups after having seen the patient in surgery; alternatively the patient could request a telephone consultation rather than a face-to-face appointment. Typically, there were only a limited number of telephone consultation appointment slots. However, there were still some surgeries that didn't offer either telephone triage or consultations, only face-to-face appointments.

There were also some practices that had already adopted the 'total triage' system, whereby *any* request for a face-to-face appointment would result in contact via the phone first. Many patients at these surgeries who had used the phone successfully would not be seen at all. The evidence at the time also indicated that at least 50% of patients did not require a face-to-face interaction following a telephone assessment. It was considered safe to deal with patients over the phone when they reviewed the reason for the call, the outcome and the subsequent need for further assessment after the phone call. *These surgeries were at a huge advantage when the pandemic hit, as they were used to caring for patients over the phone on a much larger scale.*

1.1.2   Use of the phone during the pandemic

With the advent of the pandemic, all healthcare services were forced to adopt the telephone as a means of caring for patients. In primary care, every surgery had to use the phone to deal with every request for an appointment. Clinicians who had never done telephone triage before were now having to do it and on a scale no one had envisaged. Many clinicians had never had any formal training and the stress they were put under must have been unimaginable.

They realised several things at once about telephone triage:

- It's extremely difficult, given the lack of visual cues and inability to examine directly

- It's a high-risk area

- It's a clinical specialty in its own right, requiring expertise and training

- It can be terrifying.

However, they also realised other things:

- It can be rewarding

- Patients may prefer it

- It's safer when physical contact can put both patient and clinician at additional risk

- It can be quicker and so more patients can be dealt with in each session.

1.1.3 Post-pandemic use of the phone

After we no longer had to worry as much about everyone's safety due to physical contact as we had during the pandemic, some surgeries immediately stopped offering telephone care and reverted to face-to-face appointments. Other surgeries, however, have continued to use the phone as the first point of contact. They've found it enormously beneficial for patients and staff alike and will continue to use the telephone – no matter what happens!

> **Key point**
>
> ***It is important to clarify that telephone triage or consultations only refer to calls where there is a clinical assessment of symptoms.*** Calls that should therefore not be considered a consultation nor a triage for the purpose of this book include, for example, requests for repeat sick notes, giving normal test results, repeat prescription requests or requests for letters/forms for insurance purposes or legal matters.

1.2 Telephone triage versus telephone consultations

Interestingly, the lines between telephone triage and telephone consultations were beginning to blur during the pandemic... patients simply had to be assessed over the phone before anyone was seen, but let's look at this in more detail.

Many clinicians would argue that telephone triage and telephone consultations are different and that they have a different purpose. As we've already discussed, prior to the pandemic, these terms were used to distinguish between either same-day/urgent demand (triage) and routine work (consultations). The clinicians doing 'triage' were often the duty doctor (but not always, because it could be a nurse, paramedic, pharmacist or physician associate), whilst 'consultations' were usually with the GP or a nurse only and were not considered urgent. A triage call was expected to be quick (I have seen only 3 minutes allocated to triage calls), but a telephone consultation is believed to be a fuller interaction, requiring more time (usually 10 minutes).

In my humble opinion, however, I consider telephone triage and telephone consultations to be one and the same thing – an assessment of symptoms over the phone.

The actions of the clinician are essentially the same on either a triage call or a consultation – you want to find out what the symptoms are, or how the patient is, and then decide what they need. They could need a face-to-face appointment, self-care advice or referral elsewhere, but the aim of either type of call is to determine whether the care needed can be delivered over the phone or not. Every triage can result in either a face-to-face appointment or self-care and, likewise, every consultation can result in either a face-to-face appointment or self-care. So, what's the difference once we remove the 'system' from the picture?

Also, I firmly believe that what you name these calls (a triage or a consultation) can impact on your decision-making.

- Triage calls are expected to be quick, whereas a consultation implies a more in-depth assessment but, unsurprisingly, if you want a call to be quick, it usually is. A triage call also usually leads to a face-to-face appointment, because you will be focused on getting the call done as quickly as possible and may prematurely jump to the conclusion that you need to see the patient. Asking more questions will take more time and, if you do decide you need to see the patient anyway, surely that's wasted time? Isn't it quicker just to see them? If that is the case, why bother doing any telephone triage? You may as well just see every patient.

- Telephone triage has an inbuilt assumption that the patient will be seen face-to-face and that the reason for the call is simply to assess priority – you have prejudged the outcome already, rather than assessed whether the patient actually needs to be seen. One of the biggest mistakes you can make is to prejudge the call or the outcome. It closes the mind off to possible diagnoses and can cause significant distress to you or your caller if you misjudge either the nature of the call, or the advice you are going to give.

- Consultation calls, where you give yourself a bit more time, lead to face-to-face appointments much less often, because you've undertaken a more thorough assessment and are therefore more confident when deciding that a patient can wait until later to be seen. You are also more likely to consider advising them that they can manage their healthcare problem themselves and not be seen at all (with clear guidance on what to look out for and when to call back) – if you give yourself the time to do that thorough assessment in the first place.

1.3 What would a triage call look like compared to a consultation?

This is a typical example of a 'triage call' that had been added as an emergency, where the patient told the receptionist they were experiencing chest pain. The duty doctor, well versed in telephone triage, didn't rush the call:

Clinician: *"I hear you have some pain in your chest?"*

Patient: *"Yes, doctor, it's really sore"*

Clinician: *"Do you have any other symptoms at all?"*

Patient: *"No, just this pain"*

Clinician: *"Are you sure? Anything like breathlessness, feeling sick, feeling faint?"*

Patient: *"No nothing like that, just the pain"*

Clinician: *"How are you feeling in yourself?"*

Patient: *"Fine, just a bit sore in my arms"*

Clinician: *"Is the pain going down your arms from your chest?"*

Patient: *"No, my arms have been sore for a couple of days now, but this pain just started this morning"*

Clinician: *"How would describe the pain in your chest? Does it feel like someone is sitting on your chest?"*

Patient: *"No, it's just uncomfortable on the right side, it's worse when I lift something"*

Clinician: *"You're normally fit and well aren't you? No other healthcare problems, I see from your notes."*

Patient: *"Yes that's right, but I became so unfit and put on so much weight that I've started going to the gym."*

Clinician: *"Have you been to the gym today?"*

Patient: *"Yes, I try to go first thing as it's usually a bit quieter and you can get on the weights easily"*

Clinician: *"Have you been lifting weights then?"*

Patient: *"Yeah, I've been really pleased with my progress, a new personal best today!"*

Clinician: *"Did you have this pain before you started lifting weights?"*

Patient: *"Ummm... no, not really. Well, I have had the pain in my arms before but not in my chest... that's why I rang."*

After a few more questions, the GP was able to rule out any kind of a cardiac incident and give advice on managing what turned out to be a musculoskeletal condition and not an emergency!

Now let's look at a call that was added as a telephone consultation for the nurse – a female patient had called requesting an appointment for a 'water infection'. The call was left for several hours before the nurse phoned the patient, because the receptionist didn't think it was urgent. This is what happened when the nurse spoke to the patient:

Nurse: *"Hello, I hear you have a water infection?"*

Patient: *"Yes I think so, but I feel awful"*

Nurse: *"Oh, I'm sorry to hear that. What's been happening?"*

Patient: *"Well, it started about a week ago. I had to go to the toilet all the time. I tried some of those sachets you can buy in the chemist, but it didn't really help. Now there's bits of blood in the toilet and I have this terrible pain."*

Nurse: *"Pain when you pass urine?"*

Patient: *"No, pain in my stomach and my back as well now"*

Nurse: *"In your stomach? Do you mean above your tummy button or near the pubic area?"*

Patient: *"My lower tummy"*

Nurse: *"And in your back you say? Any other symptoms or things you've noticed?"*

Patient: *"I can't get warm, but my husband says he can warm his hands on me!"*

Nurse: *"How much blood have you noticed?"*

Patient: *"It started last night as little flecks but this morning it was small clots. That's why I rang. I mentioned the blood to the receptionist."*

The receptionist hadn't picked up on the blood and, when hearing 'water infection', assumed it wasn't urgent. The patient needed an immediate face-to-face assessment and treatment for what had been originally considered a 'routine' condition and suitable for a telephone consultation.

Any call can result in an outcome you hadn't expected despite it being classed as a triage or a consultation, but the actions of both clinicians here were essentially the same – find out what the problem is and take the appropriate action. Do not prejudge the outcome because one call is an emergency triage and the other is a routine consultation.

> **Take-home message**
>
> Telephone triage and telephone consultations should be thought of as the same thing – you should never prejudge the call or the outcome based on what you call them.

Chapter 2
Things that affect your decision-making

After listening to thousands of calls in my career, I realised that there were several factors, or variables, that seem to influence the outcome of calls. This chapter describes the most common of these variables.

2.1 Operational capacity

The biggest driver which seemed to foretell whether a patient was seen (and how) appeared to be due to *operational capacity*. Put simply, if there was an appointment or slot available in either a surgery or centre, or if a home visit was possible, the patient was more likely to be seen. Once operational capacity has diminished or disappeared altogether, the triager will do their best to avoid arranging a face-to-face appointment for that session and try to deliver a 'watch and wait' outcome (sometimes hoping this means another service further down the line will pick the patient up). When services become overstretched, self-care advice seems more common, with clear instructions on when to call back if things change or worsen.

To avoid this, it is best to approach every call as if there is no capacity to see the patient; this applies even if it's the first call of the day and you have face-to-face appointments available! Ultimately, if a patient really needs to be seen they will be, it's just a matter of where/how, but if you have an appointment available you are more likely to use it. It never ceases to amaze me how outcomes change once there are operational restrictions in place, or during a pandemic where face-to-face encounters had to be avoided as much as possible for everyone's safety!

Example

Prior to the first lockdown in March 2020, I was asked to do a one-to-one training session with a GP whose conversion rate of seeing patients following a telephone call was 60–70% (as I said in *Chapter 1*, the evidence at the time suggested 30–50% conversion was safe). Their phone calls were quite long and yet they still resulted in an appointment being made two-thirds of the time. Despite my feedback, they said that they didn't think they would change that much, because they believed they were practising appropriately and safely. After a few months of lockdown, I asked how this GP had managed and I was told their conversion rates had reduced to 10%! Were they still safe? I can only hope so, but this was not an unusual conversion rate at the height of the pandemic. The key here is that the GP had been forced to think and act differently by dreadful circumstances, but I believe they weren't alone! The pandemic certainly changed opinion (and outcomes) and it is important to appreciate what can be achieved over the phone.

2.2 Who is going to see the patient?

The next variable to influence decision-making seemed to be dependent on *who is going to see the patient*. If the triager was able to book the patient in to be seen by themselves, and therefore affecting their own workload, they were more likely to arrange to see patients. If the patient was going to be passed to another colleague (and someone who was known by the triager) they were protective of the receiving clinician's workload and didn't want to pass on unnecessary work. The triager also has their own professional reputation to maintain and wouldn't want the receiving clinician to think 'that was a waste of my time', if they referred a patient on. Conversely, if there is no professional relationship between triager and receiving clinician, it can often result in very 'soft' triage, whereby excessive face-to-face appointments are given, as the triager is not worried about the workload they are passing to an unknown colleague.

Example

A GP complained that her duty doctor morning list was becoming intolerable, and she wanted the surgery to stop doing telephone triage. The duty doctor was expected to do the triage and would then have to see the patient themselves if a face-to-face appointment was necessary. When this was examined, including the outcomes, it wasn't that the list was overly long (it was the same as her colleagues'), but the GP was seeing almost all the patients she spoke to on the phone. Conversely, her colleagues were only seeing 30–40% of the patients that they triaged. When asked why she felt she needed to see so many of the patients she spoke to on the phone, she admitted she lacked confidence in telephone assessments and was nervous of not seeing patients and so missing something. She also admitted she didn't think it was an issue, because it was her own list that was being affected.

2.3 Patient or caller demand

The ***patient or caller demand*** can also influence our decision-making. If you have someone who demands to be seen (and there is a difference between a demand and an expectation which we will look at later in *Section 11.4*), or a parent who is extremely anxious and insists that you see their child, it is a rare clinician who would decline. My advice would be that if you realise that no matter what you say or do, the caller will not change their original demand, decide to say yes or no quickly and don't waste time trying to change their mind (assuming you will only do what is clinically safe, of course). It is also safer for a clinician to say no to an inappropriate demand over the phone (such as a demand for opiates) than when the patient is in front of them.

Example

A parent made it very clear at the beginning of a call that they wanted their child to be seen (for something quite minor). The GP made doubly sure about the symptoms and there didn't seem to be any risk to the child, but the parent was insistent. The GP realised that it would be a total waste of time to carry out more of an assessment on the phone and that the parent would not accept self-care measures, so they arranged a face-to-face appointment for the child – but not urgently.

2.4 Your own experiences

Next, your own *experiences* will obviously affect your decision-making. If you have ever misdiagnosed something, or had an adverse outcome following an assessment, you will naturally be more cautious with similar types of calls or patients. Once you realise that no matter how much time you take to check everything, you will always want to see the patient because you dare not do otherwise, I would advise that you simply acknowledge this and don't waste too much time on the phone, since it won't make a difference to your decision to see them face-to-face.

Example

A GP once told me that he started doing his telephone calls at the end of surgery. Unfortunately, he also seemed to want to see most of the patients after speaking to them on the phone. This meant that his surgery was regularly extended, and he would also do home visits late into the evening if patients couldn't get into the surgery. I was really concerned that he would quickly burn out if he continued this level of work, so asked him why he couldn't delegate some of the triage, or perhaps look at seeing fewer patients. He told me that he had missed something once on a phone call because he felt he'd rushed it, and the patient had come to harm as a result. So, by doing his calls at the end of the day he could take more time and it was only his workload that was affected. My advice was to see additional patients at the end of surgery and stop doing telephone triage, because no one was benefiting – it was simply increasing workload and stress.

2.5 Personality traits or habits

Finally, your own *personality traits or habits* can influence you.

- If you are a morning person or a night owl you will find your approach to calls can be different; some people think more quickly and clearly at different times of the day.

- You may have things happening at home that are making you more tired or stressed than usual.

- Some clinicians prefer to see a patient at the end of the day, rather than go home and worry about them. Others may try to give self-care advice rather than see the patient face-to-face at the end of the session, or perhaps they have another commitment that they don't want to miss so try to give a routine appointment in the future rather than squeeze in another face-to-face contact.

Dealing with patients over the phone, whereby you have a reduced ability to actually see what's happening or carry out an examination personally, is naturally a higher risk area of work, so you need to be more aware of your own mindset or functionality when you are under stress, tired or simply having a bad day! By its very nature telephone work is difficult, but having poor self-awareness can compound the difficulties.

Example

When looking at the outcomes of a team of nurses, I found that one nurse had consistently more face-to-face appointments at the end of the day than at the beginning. I assumed it was because she was being overly cautious and perhaps knew she was more tired than at the beginning of her shift, and therefore she was nervous of not seeing a patient in case she missed something. When I spoke to her, however, she said it was because it was quicker to arrange face-to-face appointments than to do a proper telephone triage – which meant she was able to pick her child up from nursery on time!

Take-home message

You need self-awareness when making your decisions. Before you offer your advice as to the outcome (be that a face-to-face appointment with a GP, nurse, pharmacist, etc.), be honest with yourself about why you are doing what you are doing. It should always be clinical need first – if a patient needs to be seen they should be seen, but if they don't need to be seen, why see them?

Chapter 3
The purpose of telephone assessments

Key points

Having a true understanding of what you are trying to achieve in a phone call or the purpose of the assessment is crucial:

- The primary aim is to determine whether a patient needs to be seen or whether their problem/request can be managed on the phone – it's **not always** about diagnosing the patient (this can be done later if you are going to see them)
- If a patient does need to be seen, you must consider how quickly and by whom
- The caller should leave the phone call satisfied with the interaction and accept your advice/outcome

3.1 The primary aim is to decide if the patient needs to be seen

Really understanding what we are trying to achieve during telephone assessment is crucial. It is primarily about assessing whether or not a patient needs to be seen, rather than making a diagnosis. However, I have witnessed many calls going on too long because the clinician was determined to make sure that they had the correct diagnosis, even though it wasn't going to change the fact that the patient needed to be seen. Whether or not the diagnosis was correct was not going to change the fact that the patient needed further face-to-face assessment. This wastes time on the phone and it can put the patient in more danger if the phone call continues when the patient needs urgent medical attention.

Once you have decided a patient needs to be seen, consider ending the call quickly if you know the diagnosis will not change the outcome. One of the most common reasons clinicians decide they need training in telephone assessment is because they are struggling to manage their time effectively or efficiently. In my experience, their calls are overly long and, when combined with a high conversion rate of phone calls to face-to-face appointments, telephone assessments have increased their workload. When they start to appreciate that once an outcome has been reached (and it can sometimes be after the first question) they should have the confidence to finish the call quickly, then they can start to use their time more effectively. Occasionally more questions are required to decide on time frame (priority), or who should see the patient (see *Section 4.2*), but these do not need to take long.

It is important to stress that I am not advocating avoiding diagnosis over the phone, but that without physical examination or confirmation, diagnosis should not be your primary aim. Each call will usually require that you reach a working or differential diagnosis on which to base your decision-making. However, avoid continuing to ask questions to try to confirm the diagnosis if you know it's not going to change your outcome of a face-to-face appointment. Those additional questions and the final diagnosis can be left to the clinician who sees the patient (see the call transcript below).

The following example is part of the transcript from a call taken at 10.30 pm by a very experienced GP. The patient was a 41-year-old woman who sounded distressed and in significant pain as soon as she spoke to the GP. This is only the first part of the call, as the remaining part of the call took an additional 5 minutes (a total of 9 minutes):

Clinician: *"How can we help?"*

Patient: *"I've got right bad pains in me ribs on't right hand side, and all in my chest and back and I'm having trouble in breathing and I feel as if I'm going to pass out"*

Clinician: *"Oh dear, OK and when did they start?"*

Patient: *"Started about 7, but they've got a lot worse since"*

Clinician: *"OK so around 7 o'clock this evening? Um, um have they been there constantly throughout the evening?"*

Patient: *"Yeah, it's just got a lot worse"*

Clinician: *"OK. Um, what's made them get worse, anything you know?"*

Patient: *"I've no idea… I can't hardly walk now, to get upstairs."*

Clinician: *"Oh dear. OK and, um, your breathing, how is that?"*

Patient: *"I'm having trouble in breathing"*

Clinician: *"You are, OK in what way?"*

Patient: *"I'm just finding it hard to breathe"*

Clinician: *"And have you ever had problems like this before?"*

Patient: *"No"*

Clinician: *"And if you take a deep breath in for me, how does that feel?"*

Patient: *"It hurts right bad"*

Clinician: *"And where does it hurt?"*

Patient: *"All over my chest and my back and me side"*

Clinician: *"So all over the right side of chest?"*

Patient: *"Yeah"*

Clinician: *"Back and side, OK?"*

Patient: *"Yeah"*

Clinician: *"Any injury there at all?"*

Patient: *"No"*

Clinician: *"OK. Have you been coughing at all?"*

Patient: *"No"*

Clinician: *"OK and this, has this just come on like this?"*

Patient: *"Yeah"*

Clinician: *"Sort of fairly sudden onset?"*

Patient: *"Yeah"*

Clinician: *"OK. Have you had any swelling or pain in your calves at all?"*

Patient: *"Not as far as I know, no"*

Clinician: *"And are you otherwise well?"*

Patient: *"I've got asthma and coeliac's disease"*

Clinician: *"OK and have you had any operations at all recently?"*

Patient: *"No"*

Clinician: *"Any recent flights or travel?"*

Patient: *"No"*

Clinician: *"Or been immobilised, plaster of Paris, anything like that?"*

Patient leaves the phone and her husband comes on

Husband: *"Hello she's had to go; she's going to be sick"*

Clinician: *"Oh dear, OK, alright"*

Husband: *"It'll be third time she's been sick"*

Clinician: *"She's been sick 3 times?"*

Husband: *"Yes"*

Clinician: *"Has she had anything for this... for the pain at all?"*

Husband: *"Not as far as I know, I don't think she's taken... she may have taken a couple of paracetamol earlier on"*

Clinician: *"Did they have any effect?"*

Husband: *"I don't think they had"*

Clinician: *"No, OK well it is a bit of a concern. Now, I was just asking Gillian whether she'd had any travel or operations or been immobilised in any way?"*

Husband: *"How do you mean?"*

Clinician: *"Well, like a plaster of Paris, or been in a wheelchair, or not being able to get out and about?"*

I hope you can see that the clinician is focused on trying to reach a diagnosis (in this case of a deep vein thrombosis followed by a pulmonary embolism) and we can tell that by the specific questions that are being asked. But the clinician failed to ask about any other symptoms, the type of pain or what is meant by "passing out" and generally how the patient is. The questions are about trying to reach or confirm a diagnosis rather than about what's happening to the patient. Would it make any difference if the patient had been travelling recently regarding the need for her to be seen, urgently, with these symptoms?

By asking questions about what's been happening historically, rather than what's happening at the time of the call, we can tell the clinician's primary aim is about trying to diagnose the patient rather than taking action to make sure the patient is safe. The cause of the symptoms can be determined once we know the patient is safe and receiving face-to-face care and assessment.

3.2 Who should see the patient and how quickly?

Once you know the patient needs to be seen, your next objective should be to decide on the priority, and then decide who should see the patient. I started my triaging career in the out-of-hours setting, where I was required to think in time frames for a face-to-face assessment to occur, i.e. 1, 2 or 6 hours. These standard time frames aren't compulsory within an in-hours settings, but they make me think about the strengths and weaknesses of having such restrictive time frames in which to see a patient. When deciding on a priority for a patient, I find it helpful to simply start with this question:

"How long do I think the patient could safely wait for?"

This makes me really consider more about when the patient needs to be seen, rather than what the appointment system dictates. I understand that we have to consider availability of appointments but, as stated in *Chapter 2*, the key driver should always be clinical need first. Once you are clear on when the patient should be assessed face-to-face, you can negotiate all the other dynamics such as patient choice, ability to get to a surgery/centre, transportation issues or parental compliance – my advice would always be ***don't move the goal posts***. This is especially true where children are concerned. Once you have decided a child needs to be seen, also decide within what time frame (remember *"how long do I think they could safely wait for?"*), but before you offer this to the carer, I would always have a Plan B, C or even D ready in case the carer can't or won't comply or accept your advice (this will be discussed in more detail in *Chapter 15*). With an adult, if there are no capacity issues, you can allow them to decide what to do about their own care, but stick to your advice and document it as such.

3.3 Ensure the caller is satisfied and so more likely to comply with your advice

This objective is perhaps the most important in many calls! I have encountered many clinicians who ask *"Are you happy with my advice?"*, but note that I have not suggested the caller is going to be 'happy' but have used the term 'satisfied'. I understand why clinicians think it is good to ask if the caller is 'happy', given that we are always taught to consider the ideas, concerns and expectations (ICE) of the patient, but I believe doing so doesn't always accomplish what you expect. Asking if someone is 'happy' is looking for an emotive response, whereas we actually really just want the caller to accept our advice and therefore comply with it; but we do want them to leave the phone call feeling listened to, satisfied that we did our best for them and that we provided information in terms they understood. This isn't necessarily giving them what they wanted or thought they needed, which is what would really have made them 'happy'.

If callers believe that you are truly listening to them and that you have addressed their concerns (real or otherwise), they are more inclined to 'like' you and feel that you have cared for them. If they like you, they will trust you and if they trust you, they are more likely to comply with your advice and cooperate more fully, whether by accepting your outcome or by giving you better quality information. If you get the caller onside right at the start, then it is easier to decide if someone needs to be seen and if so, how quickly and by whom – even the way you introduce yourself can have an impact (see *Chapter 10*).

Take-home message

You can make your calls more time-efficient, and also gain greater compliance from the caller, by understanding clearly what you are trying to achieve in a phone call, i.e. that diagnosis is secondary to whether the patient needs onward assessment. Considering what timescales are appropriate and deciding who should see the patient follow on. All of this is made easier by getting the caller to cooperate with you because they like you and therefore trust you.

Chapter 4
The risks of telephone assessments

Key points

Knowing where the risk areas are in telephone assessments will allow you to decide if the risks outweigh the benefits on a call-by-call basis. The following are some of the main issues to be aware of:

- **Assumptions** – be wary of assuming anything when you can't confirm it visually/physically
- **Confirmation bias** – clinicians try to confirm a predetermined diagnosis or outcome (even before they pick up the phone potentially) so all questions are designed to lead to that and are therefore introducing bias
- **Accurate information** – we have to rely on this from the caller, but when information is potentially inaccurate, it's safer to see the patient
- **Third party callers** – they can underplay or overplay what's wrong with the patient
- **Seeing patients unnecessarily** – there's a risk to the patient, other patients and clinicians when we see patients who didn't need to be seen
- **Time constraints** – these lead to inappropriate outcomes (commonly higher rates of face-to-face appointments) and can affect our tone of voice

We all know that there are significant risks when assessing patients over the phone, risks that in some cases are insurmountable. However, knowing where the risks lie on each individual call will allow the triager to decide how they want to manage those risks, because each call is unique in its risk profile. The same risk or issue on one call may not be dealt with in the same way on another call. For instance, if the clinician knows the patient well and the patient is used to managing their own healthcare, the clinician may decide not to see that patient because they are confident in both the information that has been shared and the patient's ability to cope. However, the same medical problem in another patient may result in the need to see the patient, because the risk is gauged to be higher due to a lack of knowledge of the patient and/or a lack of trust in the patient being able to manage the problem themselves.

So, let's look at some of the most common risks – but remember, you will need to decide on each call how to manage the risk.

4.1 Assumptions

I can't begin to tell you how often I have heard an assumption being made within a call, either by the clinician or the caller. When you can't confirm anything visually, you must check your understanding always matches that of the caller (see *Chapter 5* for more detail on how to do this). Body parts are notoriously miscommunicated – the elderly will often mistake chest pain for stomach pain – and so the triager must always seek to clarify where anything is on the body and shouldn't assume the caller has relayed the location accurately. Similarly, an assumption may happen when the clinician thinks the caller understood their question, especially when they receive an answer they are looking for (closed questions tend to lead the patient – see *Chapter 6*). As the saying goes, never *ASSUME* anything as it makes an ASS out of U and ME, but this is especially true in telephone assessments!

> ### Example
>
> A caller described 'lower' back pain to the GP. The GP didn't question what they meant and assumed it was in the lumbar area, as this is what is referred to clinically when we are referring to the 'lower back'. However, when the patient was seen, the pain was actually in the lower thoracic area, because the patient thought the back finished at the waist and the area below the waist was the 'bottom'.

4.2 Confirmation bias

Confirmation bias can mean slightly different things depending on the context within which it is used. In telephone assessments, it's when we have decided what's wrong with the patient and what we are going to do for them (sometimes before we even pick up the phone!), and consequently we use closed questions to lead to the diagnosis or outcome we have prejudged. In other words, the questions are designed to 'confirm' what we expect to hear rather than being open and allowing alternative options to be considered – therefore bias has come into the call. Confirmation bias more commonly occurs with patients whom we are very familiar with, and can even begin following receipt of information from non-clinical staff (see *Chapter 18*) regarding the reason for the call.

> ### Example
>
> An elderly lady reported having a 'water infection' to the receptionist, who then documented '?UTI' as the reason for the call back. The clinician asked only closed questions to 'confirm' the diagnosis of a urinary tract infection, but it later turned out that the patient had a sexually transmitted disease rather than a urinary infection. It seems reasonable not to consider an STD initially, especially in an elderly woman, but by predetermining the diagnosis and treatment based on the patient's own assumptions and the receptionist's 'diagnosis', the triager was misled and failed to ask the open questions which may have led to a correct diagnosis more quickly.

4.3 Accurate information

The ability of the caller to comprehend and to communicate effectively can have a significant impact on the success of the assessment. Some callers are simply unable to clearly express what's wrong with them or where something is on their body and sometimes there is a potential inaccuracy because the caller isn't with the patient. I am certainly not advocating giving advice about a patient's symptoms to a third party without the patient being present, but occasionally we can offer advice about care if we are confident in the information being exchanged. However, if you aren't confident about the information being given to you, or it isn't contemporaneous information and is therefore potentially inaccurate, you should consider a face-to-face outcome.

In some cases, the caller may struggle to give accurate information because they didn't witness what happened (see example below and also *Section 4.4*) or because of a language barrier. When you are unable to communicate clearly due to a language difference or a strong accent, there is the potential for misinformation or misunderstanding (see *Chapter 5*), in which case it is always safer to think about seeing the patient in order to assess them physically.

> ### Example
>
> A mother was concerned about her young child who had returned from staying with her ex-partner. She had been told the child had tripped over the night before when he had been running in the garden and had 'knocked his head a little bit'. He had reportedly been fine at the time and since, but the child had a minor bruise on the forehead and his mother thought he seemed quieter than normal and so had contacted the GP. The GP quite rightly felt that the lack of detail about

the extent of the injury, or the nature of the 'knock', warranted a face-to-face assessment. The child was fine, but caution was the best approach without accurate information from a witness about the way the injury had occurred.

4.4 Third party calls

A third party call is where someone phones on behalf of the patient. Most commonly calls that involve children will naturally be third party calls, but they can involve adults phoning on behalf of another adult, e.g. on behalf of an elderly relative. When you don't speak directly to the patient, however, you can miss a great deal from your initial assessment. For example, you won't hear how the patient breathes, whether they seem to be responding normally or how they sound in relation to their own healthcare problems, e.g. worried, distressed or unconcerned. Third party callers are notorious for overplaying symptoms (particularly with children) or, more worryingly, they may underplay what's wrong (see example below). Finally, third parties can make assumptions or miss something entirely – even more high risk when they aren't with the patient. Triaging through a third party can lead to a mistriage and therefore a misdiagnosis, so you should avoid third party calls whenever possible, and speak directly to the patient.

Example

A parent phoned about their 3-year-old child who was described as being 'under the weather', with symptoms that included a temperature, vomiting and diarrhoea. The clinician decided to see the child face-to-face after asking only a few questions but wasn't too worried because the parent seemed only mildly concerned. The clinician instructed the parent to bring the child in and said "just get here when you can". The parent arrived about 2 hours later and carried the child in because they were 'asleep'. Unfortunately, the child wasn't asleep but was actually unresponsive. The parent had no idea that the child was so unwell and the triager admitted they had been falsely reassured by the lack of concern from the parent and hadn't done an adequate assessment.

4.5 Seeing patients unnecessarily

Many clinicians will say that telephone assessments are high risk and that they prefer to see a patient because it's 'the safest thing to do'. Some would also argue that there is no risk in arranging to see a patient who didn't really need to be seen, other than perhaps a 'wasted' appointment. This isn't always true, however, because a telephone assessment may result in a patient being referred to a higher level of care, such as A&E rather than attending the surgery, or that arranging to see the patient may cause more of a time delay. There are risks we need to consider when agreeing to see a patient who doesn't need to be seen: there is a risk to the patient, a risk to other patients and a risk to the clinician.

Every time we agree to see a patient who didn't need to be seen, i.e. one we could have given self-care management advice to, we may increase future dependency and the patient's expectation that they will need to be seen again for the same problem in the future. Clinicians often protest that patients are too 'demanding' and that their expectations are unreasonable, but we must recognise that we can inadvertently contribute to this by seeing patients who didn't require a face-to-face interaction and could have been managed with phone advice only.

When we are busy seeing patients who don't really need to be seen, other patients can end up waiting much longer than is acceptable and may even be at risk due to these longer waiting times. If patients can't get an appointment when they want/need one, they may end up going to another service such as A&E when this isn't really appropriate, or they may even call for an ambulance. Either of these options means that another service is being deprived of a vital resource inappropriately.

You may wonder why there is a risk to the clinician, but any face-to-face outcome means someone has to see the patient. This in turn means we are increasing the workload either for ourselves or for someone else. Some patients make frequent but unnecessary contact and if they are going to be seen each time, clinicians can end up overworked and risking burnout. This is amplified even more when clinicians are nervous of telephone assessments and tend to have high conversion rates from a phone call to a face-to-face appointment. Finally, never forget that there can be a physical danger to seeing some patients, such as during the pandemic and with potentially violent patients (see example below).

> **Example**
>
> A triager arranged for a patient to be seen on a home visit by another GP. It was inappropriate to arrange for a home visit in the first place because the patient did not meet the criteria, but secondly, the patient had been asking for 'strong pain relief' according to the notes. On listening to the call, the patient is heard to request diazepam, but this was not recorded in the notes for the visiting doctor. When the GP arrived, she was greeted by the patient but also three 'mates' and a couple of bulldogs. The patient insisted they needed codeine and diazepam. The GP reluctantly gave in (it was probably the safest thing to do) and she was able to leave, but she should never have been put in that position because it was an obvious drug abuse situation. The triaging clinician had acted entirely against procedure and had placed the visiting GP in a very vulnerable and potentially life-threatening situation. When a triager suspects something such as inappropriate requests for medication, it is easier to say no over the phone.

4.6 Time constraints

The issue of time constraints is possibly one of the biggest risks when it comes to telephone assessments. Not having enough time is also probably one of the most common issues when it comes to this work. Being under time pressures has two major impacts:

- a premature conclusion

- our tone of voice is affected.

Premature conclusion is where the clinician jumps to an outcome too hastily because they are rushing the call. This can occur for several reasons: not enough time allocated to phone calls, too long a list of call backs, squeezing in a phone call between seeing patients, or the caller rushing the clinician to an outcome because they are in a hurry. The usual outcome when you feel the need to take a call quickly is often a face-to-face consult. Be aware of the conversion rate from phone call to face-to-face appointment when you are under time pressure. If you are going to reach a face-to-face outcome due to a lack of time to assess safely, then there is little point to doing phone calls at all – you may as well spend the time seeing your patients.

Tone of voice – unfortunately, when we are under a time constraint there is also a natural tendency for it to affect our tone. Without doing it intentionally, we can sound terse and there is a strong inclination to use only closed questions to keep control of the call – and therefore the time it takes. Together these things can alienate the caller, because they may feel rushed, not listened to or unable to express themselves. This in turn affects rapport, which then impacts on compliance. We will look at this in more detail in *Chapter 5*, but caller dissatisfaction due to insensitive or ill-chosen tonality can lead to complaints or unwillingness to accept advice.

Take-home message

There are many risks in telephone assessments, but understanding what the most common risks are will help you decide on how to manage those risks on a call-by-call basis.

Chapter 5
Telephone communication versus face-to-face communication

Key points

- An effective dialogue is a two-way exchange of information in terms both parties understand
- Miscommunication is often caused by one-way instead of two-way communication
- We can over-rely on what is being said (the words) rather than considering how it is being said (the tone)

The communication skills and techniques required for talking on the phone and assessing patients remotely are very different to those needed for a face-to-face interaction, for the obvious reason that you can't see each other. However, it's also more than a case of just getting information from your caller. It's about making sure you have really listened to the caller and understood the information they have conveyed, and checking that they have understood you.

Your ability to communicate on the phone can be dependent on your connection or rapport with the caller. As discussed in *Chapter 3*, if they feel listened to, they are more likely to like you; if they like you, they will be more inclined to trust you; if they trust you, they are more likely to comply with your advice. The relationship between a patient/carer and the clinician has always been one of trust, but when it comes to telephone communication, it's more difficult to develop that trust. Many patients/carers will have trouble accepting that you can care for, or diagnose someone, when you haven't seen them or examined them. You can face a huge barrier even before you start your assessment in cases where the caller mistrusts telephone assessments or has no experience of them.

The foundation for any telephone interaction is good communication, especially when you may be asked to make judgements about a patient's care without the interaction involving some communication with the patient directly. Even when you are speaking directly to the patient, you will always be missing the visual information that helps so many clinicians, such as the general appearance of the patient, their colour, their breathing – even the smell of a patient can help with our diagnostics. If you engage with your caller in a way that they respond to, you are more likely to get accurate and reliable information which will help you reach a mutually agreed management plan.

5.1 What is an 'effective dialogue'?

An effective dialogue means there is **an equal exchange of information that makes sense to you and the caller in terms that you both understand**. Making sure you have an effective dialogue is crucial, as it will lead to a more accurate triage and diagnosis, reduce the risk of errors and of missing vital information. There is a lot of evidence to indicate that when it comes to risk management of telephone triage, one of the biggest risks and therefore causes of complaints and untoward incidents, is in relation to issues of communication.

5.2 How do telephone conversations differ from face-to-face conversations?

There are some important differences to consider when talking to someone over the phone rather than in a face-to-face situation that can make a huge difference to how patients perceive us and how quickly we can gain their trust – or not.

5.2.1 Telephone conversations tend to be more formal in nature than face-to-face conversations

Studies have suggested that the conversation used when you can't see the other person sounds more like the language or linguistics you would associate with written text. This formality can make the interaction less personal, and it can be difficult to build a level of trust in each other when you aren't connecting on a personal level.

5.2.2 Negotiation is more difficult over the phone

Negotiation when done face-to-face utilises other physical attributes, such as reassuring nods of the head or an emphatic shaking of the head. Direct eye contact can also convey trust and confidence and, when appropriate, physical contact such as a reassuring hand on the shoulder can convey that you are 'on their side' and they can trust you. When talking on the phone you don't have any of these tools available to you, making negotiation and gaining trust much harder.

5.2.3 Silences can be perceived as lack of interest

When you are with a patient and they can see you, they can tell if you are quiet because you are doing something else, like checking results on a computer screen, or tidying equipment away. We therefore don't feel the need to fill the silences or explain them. On the phone, however, any silence can be perceived as lack of interest, which can make an already acutely stressed caller more emotive. If you have omitted some form of acknowledgement or 'filler' as they are known (e.g. "OK", "I see", "oh dear") to let the caller know you are listening to them, the caller may interpret this as "you're not listening to me" and become disengaged or even angry.

5.3 How do we really communicate effectively then?

We can never be totally sure that clear communication has occurred when it comes to telephone triage, but knowing where the greatest potential for miscommunication lies at least helps us try to reduce the risk. One of the biggest risks can be when communication becomes one-way instead of two-way. Typically, what can happen is one person can do all the talking (sending) whilst the other does all the listening (receiving). This means you aren't necessarily exchanging information in terms you both understand, as you aren't checking your understanding of the other person in the absence of being able to check it visually. Many of us are guilty of doing too much talking and not enough listening on the phone.

5.4 The elements of communication

Research published in 1967 (Mehrabian, A. and Wiener, M. Decoding of inconsistent communications. *Journal of Personality and Social Psychology*, 6(1): 109–114) suggested that when *thoughts and feelings were involved*, communication consisted of body language, tonality and words.

5.4.1 What's used to communicate face-to-face?

In Mehrabian and Wiener's study, when test subjects were asked where they derived their information from, the three elements reported within a ***face-to-face communication*** setting were:

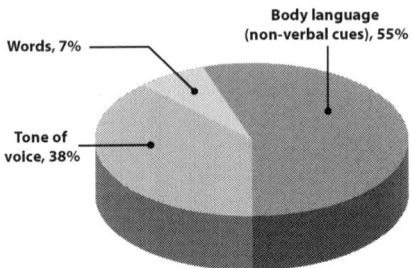

Figure 5.1 – The elements of face-to-face communication

1. **Body language** and non-verbal communication – such as nodding of the head, arm folding, eye contact, facial expressions and anything that we comprehend as a result of what we see

2. **Tone of voice** – how we say something, what inferences are used and how we choose to emphasise things

3. **The words** – what we actually say; the information that is passed verbally.

The information accrued from the following origins (see *Figure 5.1*):

55% related to visual cues, i.e. body language and facial expression

38% related to the tone or inflection in the voice

7% related to the actual content of what you say or the words used.

5.4.2   What's used to communicate on the telephone?

On the phone of course, we lose the body language that in a face-to-face situation accounts for 55% of the ability to communicate; it's replaced primarily by the tone of voice which becomes the main component of phone communication (see *Figure 5.2*).

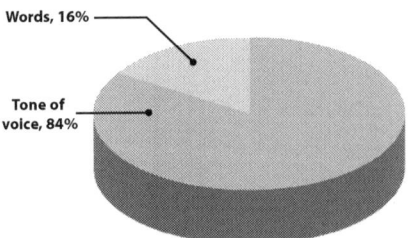

Figure 5.2 – The elements of telephone communication

As you can see, **84%** of the ability to communicate is now related directly to the tone of voice and the remaining **16%** is from the words used. A lot of your assessment, especially at the beginning, is based on how you think someone sounds, their physical state (breathless, in pain), or how you perceive they feel about something, i.e. anxious, upset, angry, etc. This isn't necessarily expressed verbally, but this information is picked up from how the caller or patient sounds (tonality).

It's not always easy to convey the importance of tonality through written information as I am attempting to do here, but think about how you would react to a parent who 'sounds' anxious: would your decision about whether or not to see a child be more affected by what the parent said, or how you thought they sounded about the situation?

5.5 What happens if information flows in only one direction?

It is very easy to have one-way flow of information during a phone call. Typically, a question is asked and answered, but neither party 'checks in' with the other to ensure they fully understand each other, by either repeating information they have received, or asking the other person to repeat the information as they have understood it. They simply accept or 'assume' they are communicating clearly.

In any phone consultation, the clinician and the caller should regularly switch from being a receiver to a sender; this means you are trying to exchange information and improves the chances of understanding each other correctly. You should ask yourself *"Did I do all the talking or all the listening, or was it an equal amount of both?"*. If it was the latter and you regularly changed from sender to receiver and back again, it's a two-way exchange of information and automatically a better consultation with less opportunity for misunderstanding or mistriage.

> ### Take-home message
>
> The key to good communication is to ensure there is a two-way exchange of information by sending and receiving information in both directions throughout the assessment. In the absence of body language, you will rely more on tonality and your caller will pay more attention to your tonality as well.

Chapter 6
Open, closed and facilitative questions – what's best?

> **Key points**
> - Most calls will use open, closed and facilitative questions
> - Facilitative questions are probably the most useful
> - Questioning techniques have to be adapted according to various issues, such as the nature of the call, the knowledge of the patient and the caller's ability to give clear information
> - The way you ask the question is as important as the question you ask
> - Be careful of multiple questions and asking the same question more than once

It's been suggested that telephone assessments are too difficult because the callers often give poor information and that leads to higher risks. It is true that callers sometimes provide poor information, but often because they were asked a 'poor' or ambiguous question.

A good consultation requires different questioning techniques at different times within the call. It's never 'one size fits all' and you must adapt your questioning technique depending on the nature of the call, your knowledge of the patient and the way in which the caller responds to the type of questions you ask.

Always remember, though, it's as much about **how** you ask the question, as it is about **what** you actually ask. Your tone of voice can convey what you are looking for, as well as the style of questions used. We will discuss the impact of tone of voice linked to a closed question in *Chapter 7*, but first let's look more closely at open, closed and facilitative questioning techniques.

6.1 Open questions

Open questions should be used as much as possible, because they prevent you from leading the caller and allow the caller to express things in their own words. It's possible to gain as much information from one open question as from several closed questions, so long as you allow your caller enough time to respond. Open questions are most useful at the beginning of the conversation and to help someone to open up if they seem quiet or reluctant to talk.

> *Advantages of open questions:*
>
> • They ask the caller to think and reflect on the situation.
> • They give the caller an opportunity to express their concerns, opinions and feelings.
> • They help the caller to realise the extent of their problem.
>
> *Disadvantages of open questions:*
>
> • You hand control of the conversation over to the caller.
> • You are expected to find a solution to their problem.
> • They can lead to pauses and a stilted conversation.

So, what does an open question look like? Here are some typical examples of open questions:

• *"What's been happening today with your pain?"*

• *"Can you describe the pain for me?"*

• *"What's worrying you exactly?"*

• *"How would you describe his colour?"*

• *"What other symptoms have you been experiencing?"*

6.2 Closed questions

There are times when closed questions are appropriate and extremely useful, such as in the case of an emergency, for summarising and to keep control when the caller keeps wandering off track.

Unfortunately, however, closed questions are more likely to be used when the clinician is busy or in a hurry. They can help get to the outcome and the end of the call far more quickly, but they can also lead your caller and give you false positives and false negatives, as can be seen in the example below:

Clinician: *"You rang about Michael? He's been vomiting."*

Father: *"Yes, it started at about 2 o'clock"*

Clinician: *"Has he got a temperature?"*

Father: *"Yes, I think so"*

Clinician: *"Have you given him any Calpol?"*

Father: *"No, I was frightened to give him anything in case he was sick again"*

Clinician: *"Has he been drinking much?"*

Father: *"No not really. Just his bottle of milk."*

Clinician: *"... and he doesn't have a rash or any tummy pain or banged his stomach at all?"*

Father: *"No"*

Clinician: *"As long as he hasn't got any pain or a rash, you could give him some Calpol and fluids and call us back if he gets any worse"*

By asking the questions in a closed way and then seeking confirmation in the same way, it's unclear if the symptoms are present. The clinician is leading the father by suggesting the child doesn't have a rash or tummy pain, rather than asking if he has had either of these symptoms. The clinician has also asked multiple closed questions, an additional risk (see *Section 6.5.1* for further information).

Advantages of closed questions:

- They are quick to answer as they require only a yes/no response, or they can be answered with a single word or short phrase.
- They help keep control of the conversation because they focus the caller.
- You can gain specific information rapidly and therefore act quickly.

Disadvantages of closed questions:

- They can lead the caller to give you incorrect information.
- They can close the caller down and prevent them spontaneously offering more information.
- They can stop the caller expressing their concerns or opinions.

Here are some closed questions to demonstrate what they look like and, as you will see, they can all be answered with 'yes' or 'no', or a very brief answer:

- *"Does he have a headache?"*

- *"Is the pain in your lower back?"*

- *"Did you say it started yesterday?"*

- *"Have you been vomiting?"*

6.3 Facilitative questions

The easiest way to understand what is meant by a facilitative question is to think of them as a multiple-choice question that provides options for the caller to choose from. In addition, it allows them to suggest an option of their own, which could be one that you hadn't considered. A facilitative question can help find out information without allowing the caller to 'ramble' (a risk with an open question) and without expressly leading (the risk with a closed question).

Advantages of facilitative questions:

- They can yield information quickly without leading the caller; especially useful in crisis situations.
- They can help you to understand what's happening by narrowing down the information by providing options.
- They can encourage the caller to expand but not hand over full control.
- The caller may come up with another solution that you hadn't thought of.

Disadvantages of facilitative questions:

- They take longer to ask than a closed question.
- They can allow the caller to take some control.

An answer to a facilitative question is typically more trustworthy or reliable than a closed question response, especially if the caller has responded with an option you hadn't suggested, rather than selected one from the options you had.

Here are some examples of facilitative questions:

- *"Is the blood bright red, brown or dark red?"*

- *"Would you describe the pain as constant or coming and going?"*

- *"If you run your hand over the rash, is it raised off the skin or is the skin flat?"*

- *"Is the sputum white, green or clear?"*

I recommend using facilitative questions whenever possible, but it's difficult to stop using closed questions when it's something you've always done. You can teach yourself to use more facilitative questions by reflecting on each call, thinking of a single closed question you used and trying to turn it into a facilitative question next time. Eventually you'll be asking more facilitative questions than closed ones.

To demonstrate once more how the techniques can differ, it's useful to see all three alongside each other, so here's an example when someone has described some bleeding:

- *"What colour is the blood?"* **(open question)**
- *"Would you describe the blood as bright red?"* **(closed question)**
- *"Is the blood bright red, dark red or pink?"* **(facilitative question)**.

6.4 The funnel technique

Using all three types of questions is a good approach in many calls and is referred to as the 'funnel technique'. This is where you begin with open and/or facilitative questions and then use closed questions to narrow down or confirm the information to reach your outcome (see *Figure 6.1*).

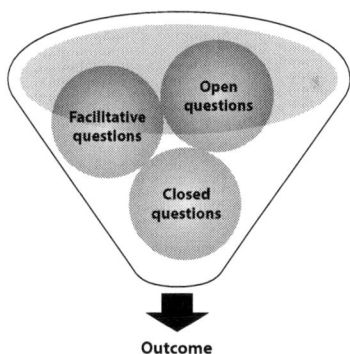

Figure 6.1 – The funnel technique.

The example below demonstrates all three techniques being used within a call. It's also a good example of using multiple closed questions in a positive way to summarise the information given:

Clinician: *"How can I help?"*

Patient: *"I've been vomiting all day"*

Clinician: *"You've been vomiting all day. Any other symptoms?"* (open question)

Patient: *"No"*

Clinician: *"How would you describe the colour of the vomit?"* (open question)

Patient: *"Quite dark"*

Clinician: *"OK, that's helpful. How many times have you vomited?"* (open question)

Patient: *"About 3 or 4 times"*

Clinician: *"Dark green or dark brown?"* (facilitative question)

Patient: *"Dark green now. It was just food, but I've not eaten all day."*

Clinician: *"Do you have any tummy pain?"* (closed question)

Patient: *"Only before I'm sick, then it goes"*

Clinician: *"So, the pain was only there before you vomited but goes straight after, it's dark green and you've vomited 3 or 4 times. You don't have any other symptoms. Is that correct?"* (closed questions to summarise).

6.5 Common pitfalls in questioning techniques

6.5.1 Asking multiple closed questions

I once had a trainee say they liked to ask multiple closed questions because it saved time. Although this may sound reasonable, there's a huge risk in this approach. For example, you might ask: *"Have you had any headaches, or a temperature or been vomiting at all"*? If the caller responds with a single 'yes' or 'no', is it in response to the headache, the vomiting, the temperature or all three? If you find yourself asking multiple questions, you will need to break them down to one question at a time to make sure your understanding of each response is correct. Let's be realistic though, how much time are you really saving by asking three questions in one compared to the greater time it would take to ask the questions individually? I suspect very little is gained time-wise but, more importantly, what's more essential, time or safety?

6.5.2 Asking questions more than once

When it comes to repeating questions, callers will often realise you are focused on something in particular. Even if you think you've been clever and asked the question in another way, the caller will know what you seem to want from them and they will give it to you – whether that's a positive or a negative response, so be careful of repeating questions too many times.

> **Take-home message**
>
> There are risks and limitations to each questioning technique, but a good call usually requires a mixture of techniques to gain accurate information. Facilitative questions are more effective in getting reliable information, compared to closed questions which can lead the caller.

Chapter 7
Examining a patient over the phone

> **Key points**
> - Only attempt asking the patient to self-examine when you are confident that you are exchanging information accurately
> - You can teach yourself to help callers/patients to 'self-examine'
> - Never take any symptom or clinical findings out of context of the patient's overall condition

Telephone assessments are difficult because we don't have the ability to examine the patient ourselves and therefore to confirm our diagnosis in many cases. So how much of an 'examination' can we really do without physically looking at or touching the patient?

First, let's compare face-to-face consultations with telephone consults a little further. We know from studies that the patient history alone in a face-to-face consult can lead to the final diagnosis in 70–90% of cases. What you are doing on the phone is taking a history, so 70–90% of the time we should be able to reach a diagnosis from that history alone, shouldn't we? The advantage of course when we are in front of the patient is that we can confirm our diagnosis by carrying out a physical examination, but how much of that can we do reliably on the phone?

I've found that a good way to think about this is to visualise a patient that you have seen face-to-face recently and one where you felt you had taken a history that was accurate because you were communicating effectively with each other. After taking the history, did you uncover clinical findings during the examination that you weren't expecting or did you hear, feel or see something that you were expecting given the history you took? I suspect that your examination will have confirmed what you expected to find, rather than surprised you. So, on the phone, if you are confident in the history you have taken, imagine that the patient is in front of you and decide whether there would be any real need for a clinical examination after taking the history. Would it be just to confirm your diagnosis? Are you already confident about what the problem is? If that's the case, you might consider dealing with the patient over the phone rather than seeing them or referring elsewhere if necessary. If, however, the history wasn't precise enough and therefore you are unsure what the clinical findings might be, you should be more inclined to see the patient.

7.1 Is it even an 'examination' if we haven't done it ourselves?

I would contend that it is an examination that we are asking the caller to do on our behalf. There are some fundamentals that we can often do, such as asking for temperature readings, blood pressure readings or blood sugar readings (where the appropriate equipment is available). You could also ask for pulse rates or respiration rates if you are confident in the caller's ability to measure these accurately. When it comes to a more in-depth examination that includes things such as self-palpation or asking parents to describe the appearance of a rash, it is a different level. There is one important point I'd like to make in relation to any patient self-examination: you won't be able to trust the results of any 'examination' if you don't trust the information you are sharing. *If you don't have confidence in the way you are communicating or your understanding of the caller's descriptions, there is little point in doing any kind of examination.*

7.2 How do we examine someone over the phone?

When you trust your ability to communicate with your caller and you feel it's appropriate to attempt some form of examination, I think it's worth starting the conversation with the following phrase:

> *"As we aren't in the same room, you are going to be my eyes, ears and hands."*

This phrase is a positive approach in gaining the caller's cooperation and trust in what you are about to ask them to do. The phrase *"as I can't see you"* is a more negative statement and can bring mistrust into the encounter. The caller may begin to doubt the validity of your advice, or the reason for attempting some examination on your behalf. I try to avoid saying *"I can't see you"* unless it's absolutely necessary and usually that's only when I want them to follow my instructions to get urgent care!

If you are willing to see how much you can get the caller to do on your behalf over the phone, you might be surprised at how effective it can be. One GP told me, after I had proposed patient self-examination, that she was horrified at my suggestion, but went away and reflected on it. She told me a couple of years later that it had been "a slow burner" and she is now happily asking patients to report back on self-examination with great confidence.

The best way to teach yourself to help patients to self-examine over the phone is to start by asking callers to self-examine only when you are going to see them anyway. When you do see them, ask them to show you what they did over the phone and you will be able to see how effective your instructions were. Not only that, but also how well you interpreted their response. Over time you will see how positive your self-examinations were and how well you interpreted the results. You will then gain more confidence in doing this. Alternatively, of course, you may also realise you aren't doing it very well, and so you should probably stop!

7.3 An example of self-examination – abdominal pain

Abdominal pain is notoriously difficult to assess over the phone and most of the time clinicians will want to see the patient for an in-person examination. I totally understand why this is the case, but most abdominal pains aren't investigated further unless it is recurring pain, or the patient is obviously systemically unwell. On palpation, most abdominal pains are benign, and patients are advised to keep an eye on things and return if the pain worsens or doesn't resolve.

Over time I have become more comfortable with asking patients to self-palpate their abdomen for me, but always with caution in mind and by remembering that it's not only about whether a patient gets seen, but when and by whom.

I begin by looking at the overall presentation of the patient. If they sound as if they are in severe pain and they report that they can't find a position of comfort, or that any movement aggravates the pain, I have already decided on a face-to-face outcome and it needs to happen pretty quickly. If, however, they sound normal, i.e. no outward sounds of distress and the pain is reportedly intermittent (and perhaps not even there at the time of the call), I am happier to think about self-palpation (see below for more detail on how this can be done).

Example – self-palpation of the abdomen

Clinician: *"As we aren't in the same room, you will be my eyes, ears and hands. If we were together I would want to feel your tummy, but you are going to do that for me. I'd like you to begin by lying down flat, even on the floor if that's possible. Would you be happy to do that for me?"*

If the patient is able and willing to lie down flat, it's unlikely that they would have an acute abdomen, such as peritonitis. If they say they'd rather not do that for me, as it 'hurts' more, stop the examination and ask to see them fairly soon.

If they go to lie down, however, and you hear a 'grunt' or 'moan', don't assume anything yet.

Clinician: *"That sounded uncomfortable for you – could you tell me where it was uncomfortable?"*

If the caller tells you that their pain in their abdomen was aggravated by moving, consider seeing them, but patients may respond by saying "my knees are killing me" – so never assume anything!

If the patient sounds quite well, they are willing to lie down and they weren't made more uncomfortable by doing so, then go on to ask:

Clinician: *"OK, when I ask you to, I'd like you to press firmly on the spot you said was uncomfortable for you and keep pressing until I tell you to stop. Would you be happy to do that for me?"*

If the patient declines to press on the painful area as it makes the pain worse, or they cooperate and press on the area which then increases the pain, they should be seen quickly. If they press firmly and report a mild irritation, consider seeing them, but not urgently. If they say the pain is not present on palpation I'd be more inclined to watch and wait.

With time, patience and practice, you should get more comfortable asking patients to examine themselves. *Remember though, **never take the symptoms out of context to the patient**.* How do they sound? Are symptoms present at the time of the call? Does anything make the symptoms better or worse? If the patient already sounds in pain at the time of the call and they report aggravation of that pain when they are touched or move, don't bother with any further questions, just see them.

One final point: don't forget that how you ask these questions can make a difference. Your tone can imply you are looking for a positive or negative response and a closed question such as *"Did that hurt?"* is more likely to encourage a *"yes"* in response rather than a question such as *"How did that feel?"*.

Take-home message

Self-examination is possible, but only when you and the patient are communicating effectively and you trust the information you are sharing. If there is any doubt about the accuracy of the information, consider seeing the patient.

Chapter 8
The importance of having a structure to your call

> **Key points**
> - Having a structure helps capture relevant information
> - Structure leads to increased confidence in your decision-making
> - Patients will respond more positively if you demonstrate a structured approach
> - Beware of being too inflexible when following a structure or protocol

When listening to calls, I realised how much a good call structure impacted on the quality and length of a call, as well as on the decision-making and confidence of the triager. So many calls become almost chaotic in the absence of visual information, and this chaos can then lead to important information being missed, or time being spent on unimportant or irrelevant information. Also, there is nothing worse than thinking of a question you should have asked after you have completed the call, but this isn't uncommon when a call has lacked focus and organisation. A disordered approach leads to confusion and lack of assertion, which can then lead to mistrust on the part of the clinician as well as the caller.

Just as in a conventional face-to-face consultation, a good call structure or 'model' allows you to think more clearly, improves your information-gathering process and ***increases your confidence***. This is vital to allow you to practise effectively and without the constant worry of "should I have seen them?" when you close a call with self-care management. Lack of confidence when doing telephone assessments is one of the main reasons so many clinicians sign onto my training courses. I have encountered clinicians who have undertaken telephone work for decades and yet they still lack self-assurance in their decision-making and so see patients who could have been helped over the phone alone.

A simple structure is to have three clear stages:

- Beginning – the introduction (see *Chapter 10* for full details)

- Middle – the history-taking (see *Chapter 11* for full details)

- End – where you agree on a management plan (see *Chapter 12* for full details).

By following the three basic steps (in the thorough way outlined in the individual chapters) when taking a call, we should ensure we are addressing the issues in order and with enough detail so that we can close the call knowing we have tackled the problem and the patient's concerns adequately and safely.

It's not only about understanding the three stages of a call, but also about completing the stages in order. Clinicians commonly mix up the stages of a call, offering the outcome or diagnosis at the wrong time (see example below) or asking more questions after agreeing to see the patient, for instance. What if you change your mind about either the diagnosis or the outcome? The caller will lose confidence in you, and you might doubt yourself if you are constantly backtracking.

Example of poor call structure

Clinician: *"What's the problem?"*

Parent: *"My son seems to have developed some spots on his tummy, with blisters. He's got a bit of a temperature and he's just not himself."*

Clinician: *"It sounds like it could be chickenpox"*

In this example, the clinician has revealed what they believe to be the diagnosis, but before they have carried out a full assessment. That's not to say that it doesn't seem a reasonable diagnosis, but by offering the outcome or diagnosis prematurely, it can affect the questions subsequently asked and lead to confirmation bias (as discussed in *Section 4.2*). The diagnosis is part of the third stage of a call (the management plan) and yet it has been spoken about before stage 2 (the information-gathering stage) has been completed.

My call methodology can be applied to any type of call or patient. My approach to the information-gathering stage (stage 2) is a generic one, rather than demonstrating the specific questions that you would find in condition-specific telephone triage protocols. Condition-specific protocols, as well as clinical decision support systems such as the one used by NHS 111, provide precise detail related to the symptoms being assessed. However, whether it is my structure, your own structure or one that has been provided for you, be careful of adhering too strictly to a structure; each call must be treated individually because patients aren't all the same in either their answers or presentations. Protocols can be too inflexible or insufficient for some cases, so always be mindful that a structure is there to guide your decision-making. Ultimately, you may have to consider asking questions that a protocol hasn't suggested or interpret the answers differently depending on other influences, such how the patient sounds versus what they tell you.

Take-home message

Develop a structure that works for you and your own style of assessment, but make sure you have a definitive structure for your calls to allow you to capture relevant information and to close the call with confidence. Any structure, however, should be one that can be adapted to different patients and presentations.

Chapter 9
Preparing to take a call

> **Key points**
>
> - Allow adequate time for taking calls
> - Review the reason for the contact **but** anticipate that it might be incorrect, so don't be disconcerted if it's wrong
> - Think about when is the best time to read the patient's notes
> - Smile as you introduce yourself – it can make a difference even though the patient can't see you

The triage process starts before you even speak to the patient, because there are some basic things you need to do to prepare yourself to take a call.

9.1 Make sure you have adequate time

I know this can be more easily said than done, but remember the impact of time constraints (see *Section 4.6*). By having to take a call quickly due to time constraints, decision-making and tonality are affected, so always try to give yourself adequate time to take a call.

9.2 Review the reason for the contact

Hopefully you will have some knowledge of the reason for the contact if the call is initiated by the patient or if it's a follow-up call, but review any notes taken by a receptionist, call handler or other clinician. However, *although you should expect that the information entered is accurate, always consider that it might not be*. Many a clinician has been caught out by assuming that the notes entered by someone else are accurate, but when they call the patient back they are asked to assess something completely different! This can happen for various reasons: the receptionist may have missed something, the caller may have withheld something or even lied to get access to the clinician, or the previous clinician may have mistriaged or documented incorrectly. By anticipating that you may hear something from the caller that isn't documented, you won't be caught out.

9.3 Decide when would be the best time to read the patient's notes

Assuming you have access to the patient's notes, consider carefully when is the most appropriate time to read them, i.e. before you speak to the patient, during the phone call itself or even after you have reached your outcome.

9.3.1 Before you speak to the patient/caller

Ideally, you will have time to read a patient's notes before ringing them, particularly if the information that you've been given about the reason for the contact indicates a less urgent issue. In this case, you may want to read the notes before picking up the phone, so that you have an idea of past medical history and maybe any social issues which may affect your decision-making, such as whether the patient lives alone, is a carer or perhaps a single parent of several children.

9.3.2 Whilst you are speaking to the patient/caller

Reading the patient's notes whilst you are talking to them is not optimal because it can be a distraction – is it safe to try to read the notes when you should be listening carefully? It may be better to put them on hold to read the notes undistracted.

9.3.3 Reading the notes after you have reached an outcome

On very rare occasions you may consider reading the notes after the call – probably only because it was an emergency, or you were worried about the safety of the patient at the time of the call. Once you've read the notes, you can always consider if it's necessary to call the caller/patient back if you discover anything that might affect the management plan.

9.4 What information should you read?

The patient's primary care notes are usually available to both in-hours and out-of-hours organisations. Clinicians generally like to read the following in a patient's notes when they are unfamiliar with the patient:

- the past medical history (PMH)
- the medications the patient is taking

- the summarised history

- the last few consultations (especially with children).

If the clinician knows the patient well, it is possible to just look at the last consultation before speaking to the patient. But when assessing children, it is particularly important to check several of the most recent consultations to make sure that you aren't missing any safeguarding issues, e.g. several attendances/contacts but via a variety of services, which could indicate that the carer is trying to hide that they have been seen multiple times.

9.5 Smile as you introduce yourself

We will talk about what to say when you introduce yourself in *Chapter 10*, but whatever you choose to say and do, I would highly recommend you smile as you begin introductions. We know that you can hear a smile in someone's voice and smiling makes you sound friendlier and interested – if you don't believe me, just give it a try! One GP reported recently that since he began to smile as he introduced himself he hadn't had an aggressive caller in over 2 years. Your tone of voice replaces the physical smile or handshake you might use in person, so it must sound welcoming, confident and helpful.

> **Take-home message**
>
> Your call structure begins before you even speak to the caller, so make the right preparations, including putting a smile on your face. Consider when is the safest time to read the patient's notes.

Chapter 10
Stage 1 of taking a call: the introduction

> **Key points**
>
> • Be careful of how and when you identify yourself
> • Ask to speak directly to the patient when appropriate and possible to do so
> • Check you have the right notes
> • Check the location of the patient

The following model is based on a clinician returning a call that a patient or carer has placed requesting a call back. If you are taking a call directly (i.e. picking up the call from cold), you can omit some of the introduction accordingly.

10.1 Be careful of identifying yourself until you know who you are talking to

The issue of when and how you identify yourself can be a contentious point. Many clinicians have expressed frustration when I suggest they need to exercise extreme caution when the patient is unknown to them and they are unaware of the social circumstances of the patient. By opening a call in the way shown below, you may betray confidentiality at least or inadvertently endanger the patient at worst:

> *"Hello, it's the Doctor/Nurse here from the surgery, can I speak to (asks for patient/caller by name) as they have asked for a call today."*

This approach assumes that because the caller has requested a call back and provided the number on which to call them, it's a reasonable way to begin the call. However, indemnity companies are warning clinicians of the dangers of identifying yourself as a healthcare professional before clarifying who you are talking to. They suggest that legally it could be argued that the implied consent of using a number in the patient's notes does not extend to identifying yourself as a clinician, or indicating that you are ringing from the practice / out-of-hours service, to whoever answers the phone. The patient may not want anyone else to know they had requested a call back and therefore you could be breaching confidentiality to say so.

The receptionist can help in some cases (see *Chapter 17*) because they can ask for consent for you to identify yourself but, in the absence of specific consent, you may need to rethink your approach. I have been told of many cases when a breach of confidentiality has put patients at risk, but the worst case is described in the example below.

> ### Example of when a GP identified himself as a doctor before establishing the identity of the person who answered the phone
>
> A GP from an out-of-hours service rang the number left by a young female patient. The conversation began:
>
> *"Hello it's the doctor here from the out-of-hours service. Can I speak to (names the patient) because she's asked us to give her a ring this evening?"*
>
> *"I'm her father, what's this about doctor?"*
>
> The GP avoided saying anything about the reason for the call, but he was told the patient wasn't at home. The GP said he would try again later and ended the call. It transpired the patient was actually at home, but her father had answered her mobile phone. The patient was forced by her father and brother to tell them why she had contacted the service. It transpired she was concerned she might be pregnant. Unfortunately, the family believed that honour killings were acceptable in such a situation and they then murdered the girl.
>
> This chilling tale all began because the GP identified themselves as 'the doctor' and even though no confidential information was disclosed, simply saying who they were led to a tragic outcome.

Another case occurred when a female patient rang her surgery requesting a consultation. The GP knew the patient, as she had seen her before, but not particularly well. When the GP returned the call after it had been taken originally by the receptionist, the conversation was as follows:

Clinician: *"Hello, it's the doctor here. Is that Janice?"*

Patient: *"Yes, how long will you be?"*

Clinician: *"I'm sorry Janice, but if you are requesting a home visit I couldn't do that until I find out what's the problem. How can I help?"*

Patient: *"Just beep your horn when you get here"*

Clinician: *"I'm sorry, as I said, I need more information before I visit. What's been happening?"*

Patient: *"Have you got the right address?"*

The doctor told me she was about to consider disconnecting as this was all so strange, but then she thought perhaps there was more to this:

Clinician: *"Just answer yes or no Janice, are you in danger?"*

Patient: *"Yes, that's right"*

The patient was in an abusive relationship and had called the GP for help but wasn't able to state that outright. So, she had prepared a story for her abusive partner about ringing for a taxi so that if he overheard the conversation, or questioned who had been ringing her, she would be able to say it was about arranging a taxi. Due to the quick thinking of the GP, she was able to send help, but if the partner had answered the phone, I doubt that she would have been given access to the patient after her introduction.

These are extreme and rare cases and ones I hope you will never encounter, but they highlight that an alternative approach may be safer. As such, it is better in your introduction to ask for the caller/patient first and then wait to see what kind of a response you get. I have found the following examples work:

Clinician: *"Can I speak to .... (names patient/caller) please?"*

Person who answers phone: *"Who's calling?"*

Clinician: *"......... (names patient/caller) asked me to give them a ring today. Are they available?"*

Person who answers phone: *"But who are you?"*

Clinician: *"I am really sorry, I don't mean to sound mysterious, but they have placed a call today and asked for a call back. Are they available?"*

Another approach could be:

Clinician: *"Can I speak to .... (names patient/caller) please?"*

Person who answers phone: *"Who are you?"*

Clinician: *"My name is .... (provides name without using title of doctor or indicating that they are a nurse). They asked me to give them a ring today. Are they available?"*

When put in contact with the patient/caller, the clinician responds:

"Hello, it's Dr ...../ Nurse..... here. How can I help?" (This establishes professional title once you know that you are talking to the patient.)

I mentioned previously that when you know your patient and their social circumstances very well, you can usually be confident that there isn't a risk in identifying yourself up front. There is also another set of circumstances in which it is better to ignore this cautious approach and that's when you are concerned a patient's life or limb may be at risk.

If you have information about the patient that indicates a potential emergency, such as 'chest pain', 'fitting uncontrollably' or 'not breathing very well', then you should get access to the caller or patient who needs help as quickly as possible and worry about your introduction later. So in this case, I would begin with *"Hello, this is Dr/Nurse........ Can I speak to .... (names patient) please?"*. You can defend your actions because the patient was potentially at risk and gaining access to the patient is your primary concern. If you unwittingly breach confidentiality, you can only apologise and ask that this is disregarded when you are concerned for the patient's safety.

Many clinicians feel strongly that this approach of withholding your identity until you know who you are talking to is overly cautious and can in fact get in the way of expediting the phone call. It is of course up to you as an autonomous practitioner to decide on what is right for you and your patient. But underpinning this advice is the need to always protect confidentiality, except in the case of an emergency when confidentiality is secondary to safety.

10.2 Ask to speak directly to the patient

As discussed in *Chapter 3*, there are risks associated with assessing a patient through a third party, but many calls are placed by a third party even when it isn't necessary; in other words, the patient is present, but someone has rung on their behalf. If this is the case, I would encourage you to try to speak directly to the patient if at all possible. Don't be put off by the other person saying, *"they want me to talk for them"*. I often say, *"it will only be for a second and they can pass the phone back at any time"* and then find I can complete the assessment directly with the patient. It isn't always possible or appropriate to speak directly to the patient, but when there is no alternative but to assess using the third party, don't forget the risks of doing so and try to minimise those risks as much as possible.

10.3 Check the demographics of the patient

Mistakes can be made when retrieving the patient's notes, so always check the demographics of the patient to ensure you have the correct notes – especially when the patient isn't known to you. As a minimum I would suggest you ask for the date of birth (DOB) and the postcode of the patient.

10.4 Check the location of the patient

If you are calling a patient on a mobile phone, it's good practice to check on their physical location just in case it is an emergency and you get cut off, or in case you need to send an ambulance.

> **Take-home message**
>
> Within the introduction of a call, you should have an awareness of confidentiality versus safety and speak directly to the patient when appropriate and possible.

Chapter 11
Stage 2 of taking a call: taking a history

> ### Key points
> - Start the consultation with an open question
> - Confirm what the patient is doing to establish their immediate condition
> - If appropriate, consider asking how the patient seems to a third party to get a better understanding of their condition
> - Establish the caller's agenda to help manage expectations
> - Consider speaking directly to children to get your own impression of how they are
> - Ascertain the history of the symptoms
> - Ascertain the patient's history

11.1 Start the consultation with an open question

Although you may have been given the reason for the contact, by a receptionist for instance, it's always good practice to begin the consultation with an open question to determine the reason for the call directly from the caller/patient. By doing this, you will avoid giving the caller any incorrect information documented by the receptionist (see *Section 9.2*) and thereby starting the conversation negatively. I like to use one of the following phrases:

- *"How can I help you today?"*

- *"You rang about your son/daughter, what can I do to help?"*

- *"What's been happening?"*

I try to avoid saying *"what's the problem?"* because I feel it's a negative start to the conversation, but many clinicians do like to use this statement. Find something that you are comfortable with.

Remember though, you must be ready for *"do I have to go through it all again?"*. One way of handling this would be to use phrases like *"If you don't mind. I've got all the information in front of me that you gave to* (state the role of previous encounter, e.g. the receptionist), *but it's much safer if I can hear it from you again in your own words"*. Note the word 'safer' and not 'better', as this brings in the clinical aspect and stops the caller thinking 'better for whom?'.

Give the caller enough time to respond (usually 30–60 seconds is enough) and listen carefully. Try to resist the urge to interrupt, and focus completely on what they are saying rather than on the questions you want to ask. The way the caller expresses what the problem is will give you a good insight into how they feel about it and what their concerns are. Don't forget to repeat the reason for the call back to the caller to make sure you understand exactly what's happening and that you are about to assess the right thing – especially if there are multiple symptoms.

11.2 Confirm what the patient is doing

Once you have a clear idea of the reason for the contact, make sure you understand what the patient is doing at the time of the call. If the patient is an adult and they are at work, it's tempting to think "well it can't be that bad then if you're able to go to work", but for some patients that may not be fair or accurate. Many people today are on zero-hours contracts and not going to work means no income, so they will struggle into work when perhaps they shouldn't have done so. By asking what work they do, however, you will get a better impression of how ill someone is if they are able to carry out their normal activities.

You should also be mindful of the environment the caller may be in, i.e. whether it is suitable for an open discussion. A teenager may be reluctant to speak openly in front of parents, for instance, or the patient may be travelling. I once had a patient, however, who told me she was shopping in a supermarket, but she was still more than happy to discuss her very personal problem with me whilst doing so!

11.3 How does the patient seem to a third party?

If there is a third party present, they can be very useful in determining how well or unwell a patient is if you don't have prior knowledge about the patient, or are not sure that you fully trust the history given by the patient. If the patient gives you permission, it may be appropriate to ask the third party how the patient generally seems to them. Remember not to use phrases that could lead them, such as *"do they look pale?"* but instead ask how they look, or ask whether they look different to their usual self. When drug or alcohol use is involved, patients may deny what they have taken whilst the third party will often give you a more accurate account.

Also, with mental health illness, the third party may know what an acute situation is or what is normal for the patient, even though it may sound serious to you. If you have a parent who expresses grave concern about their child by saying something like *"I've never seen them like this before in my life"*, it's a very difficult level of anxiety to overcome, so you are probably going to see the child anyway, therefore little more assessment is usually needed.

11.4 Find out the caller's agenda as soon as you can

This is probably one of the most valuable things I ever learnt as a triager – find out what the caller wants as soon as you can. Is it a demand or an expectation? Once you understand what they want from you or what their chief concern is, it will help you establish a rapport and manage the rest of the call. The examples below provide differing phrases that will help you to find out the caller's ideas, concerns and expectations. But ultimately you are trying to determine how best to approach the call so that you can address those concerns quickly, or even to decide if there is any point in continuing the call if the caller's anxiety is unsurmountable.

Example questions to discover the patient's agenda

- *"What is it you are hoping I'll be able to do for you today?"*
- *"Before we begin, do you have something in mind as to what the problem may be?"*
- *"Is there anything in particular that you are concerned or worried about?"*
- *"What is worrying you the most about this?"*
- *"You know your child best, what worries you the most?"*
- *"If you've had the pain for several days, can you tell me what made you ring today rather than yesterday? What's different today?"*

However, when you know the patient well and have found them to be unreasonably demanding (even abusive) in the past, there is often little point in beating about the bush so I may even ask *"So, what is it that you want from me today?"*.

You also have to be ready for any response to questions, such as these: *"You're the doctor, you tell me what's wrong!"* or *"I have no idea, that's why I rang you!"*. If this happens, I often respond *"OK, that's good to know, now we both have an open mind about things"* and then ask a question to get the assessment underway before they have any more opportunity to be negative.

11.5 Consider the value of speaking to children

When the patient is a child, it may be appropriate to ask to speak to them directly in the same way you would if the patient was an adult. If the child was in your clinic, you would certainly direct some of the conversation towards them and introduce yourself to them, even if they are unable to respond verbally, so why not do the same thing over the phone? However, I am not suggesting that you carry out the full assessment through the child, merely that you speak to them briefly to gain your own impression of how they sound. If you have forgotten to ask where the child is or what they are doing, by asking to speak to them you will find these things out. Hearing how the child sounds may help you to reach your outcome more quickly. For example, if they sound entirely miserable, distressed or in pain, or you can hear unusual breathing or coughing, you should probably arrange to see the child quickly. On the other hand, some parents overplay how ill their child is and, by asking to speak to them briefly, you can judge for yourself that the child is not as ill as you had been informed. If you do speak to the child, you should also document your impression in the child's notes, so that if there is a delay or denial of care and the child deteriorates, your decision will be supported by your documentation of their condition as you heard it at the time of the call. Generally, by speaking to the child directly you will probably be more reassured and more confident in managing children without the need to see them all. In the example below, it certainly helped me with the parents' expectations and subsequent management of the call.

> **Example**
>
> I once asked to speak to a 6-year-old child who, according to the mother, *"needed antibiotics for her tonsillitis"*. After gaining permission to talk to the child, I asked her where she was (I wanted to hear how her voice sounded, i.e. constricted, throaty, normal, etc.). To my surprise she answered *"Pizza Hut"*. I asked if she had eaten any pizza, to which she responded *"Yes, three bites"*. When I then spoke to the mother I said, *"As you probably heard, she told me she was in Pizza Hut; that's great. She also said she has had some pizza to eat and that's really reassuring. Now let me ask you some more questions"*.
>
> I avoided the need for a face-to-face consult, as well as antibiotics, because I was able to use the information positively and reinforce with the parent that antibiotics weren't needed at that time.
>
> She didn't call back.

11.6 Ascertain the history of the symptoms

We are now about to go into more detail about the symptom (or symptoms) the patient is experiencing, and it's important to find out all the information we need in a logical order. We also need to stay focused, so we don't waste time on irrelevant information or details that don't have any bearing on the current situation. The question, though, is what's irrelevant?

The skill in telephone triage is not to rush too quickly into the assessment before finding out what is really going on and by giving the caller the chance to mention all symptoms at the beginning of the call. Always ask *"any other symptoms?"*, or words to that effect, to make sure they haven't forgotten anything. If you are worried the caller may not realise the relevance of some symptoms, try spending more time probing about what's been happening, how they are managing to function and any other symptoms that they've noticed (all open questions), rather than a straightforward *"do you have…?"* (closed question). Just because someone hasn't mentioned something specifically, doesn't mean it isn't happening. In the event of problems or a complaint following a call, the key question that will be asked of you is *"did you make every effort to find out?"*. The poorest response you can give is *"they didn't tell me"*, unless you have allowed them plenty of opportunities to mention something, or asked enough questions to try to find out if it was an issue for them.

On some occasions you must be confident that despite the caller mentioning something that has occurred, it isn't relevant given the rest of the history and therefore you choose not to investigate it further.

The best way to stay focused is to develop a structure or template for gathering information. By concentrating on contemporaneous information first in relation to the symptoms and then on the patient's history, it means we are dealing with the safety of the patient as a priority.

So how can we take a history in a structured way? I have found the template below to be beneficial, in that it allows me to collect information about what's been happening and can be applied to adults or children of any gender.

This template is not condition-specific and won't provide enough details about each symptom. For instance, if the complaint was vomiting, the template doesn't go into detail about the colour, frequency or type of vomiting, but the clinician's critical thinking will fill in that level of information. It allows the clinician to decide for themself what specifics they need to know to assess the symptoms without getting bogged down in unnecessary detail.

Symptom history	
What is the chief complaint?	
What are the associated symptoms?	
Characteristics of chief complaint?	
Onset of chief complaint?	
Duration of chief complaint?	
Location?	
What has helped or made it worse?	

A last word of warning though – make sure you don't fall into the trap of trying to complete every section just for the sake of it or take the symptoms out of context of the patient.

Now let's look at each of these headings in more detail.

11.6.1   What is the chief complaint?

When patients have multiple symptoms, you need to decide what the chief complaint is and what you want to assess first. By taking your time to decide on the chief complaint and assessing that alone to a conclusion, you will help to streamline your assessment. Many calls become chaotic because the clinician is trying to assess multiple symptoms all at the same time, and then ends up getting bogged down in too much detail or missing key elements.

When trying to identify the chief complaint, it may seem reasonable to ask the caller what worries them most, but the caller may not realise that certain symptoms are more concerning than others. For instance, a patient may be suffering from vomiting and diarrhoea in equal measure, but they feel that the diarrhoea is the most unpleasant, so to them this may be the chief complaint. Vomiting, however, can be caused by many things and preclude a serious incident, whereas diarrhoea is less likely to predispose a life-threatening condition and tends to be more self-limiting. Therefore, vomiting should be the chief complaint.

Once you have assessed the chief complaint, if you decide a face-to-face outcome is required then you may not need to assess any other symptoms over the phone because you can do that when you see the patient. However, if assessing other symptoms might affect the urgency of your outcome, it may be useful to carry out a secondary assessment. If you decide not to see the patient after assessing the chief complaint, how much more do you need to know about the associated symptoms anyway if they were less concerning? Identifying the most serious symptom and then reaching an outcome can save you a lot of time by preventing further discussion about less significant issues.

11.6.2 What are the associated symptoms?

Although you may not need to carry out much investigation into any associated symptoms, it's still necessary to collect the information. If there are several complex symptoms and the patient sounds very unwell, you may well already have decided to see the patient and so now you just need to consider how quickly and by whom.

11.6.3 Characteristics of the chief complaint

When looking at the main symptom, you will need to find out more detail. What are the features or physiognomies of the symptom? How does the chief complaint present? For instance, if the chief complaint is abdominal pain, what type of pain is it, i.e. dull, sharp, constant or intermittent? Does it move or is it stationary? If the chief complaint is vomiting, what colour is the vomit? What type of vomiting, i.e. projectile? How often is the patient vomiting? You need specific details about the chief complaint.

At this point I find it useful to summarise the symptoms in combination with how the patient is generally, as mildly, moderately or severely unwell. If they are leaning towards severely unwell, you are likely to want to see the patient, in which case it's now about deciding how soon and by whom.

11.6.4 Onset of the chief complaint

This section of the template is self-explanatory; we are looking for a time that the chief complaint began. If there are multiple events reported, you may want to know when the first event was and when the last event occurred, so you have a clear idea of not only when it started but also how long it is since they experienced it.

11.6.5 Duration of the chief complaint

Having established whether it's a single occurrence or multiple episodes of the chief complaint, we now need to establish when the single episode started or, if there are multiple episodes, how long each episode lasted (and if it's still there at the time of the call, of course). We are trying to establish if there is any change in pattern at all. For example, with abdominal pain, if the first episode lasted 10 minutes but the latest one has been going on for over an hour, it would suggest a worsening disease progression. On the other hand, episodes that are decreasing in length may indicate a less immediate need for a face-to-face appointment and an improving situation, despite pain still being present.

11.6.6 Location of the chief complaint

This part of the template isn't always necessary to address. For example, if the chief complaint is nausea or low mood there is no specific 'location', but if the complaint is a pain or a rash, finding out its exact location is important. However, it's one of the hardest things to do over the phone. It often leads to assumptions or a misunderstanding due to a lack of clarity.

Use terms the caller will understand to identify parts of the body or, if you need to know the size of something, using coin sizes can help, e.g. the size of a 5p or 50p coin. Find a point of reference (and possibly use this point in relation to another) to get a clear description of where something is. Never take the caller's own description as being accurate – 'kidney pain' is notoriously misrepresented! You need to build your own understanding of where something is. Lay terms are always best. If you are worried about insulting the intelligence of the caller, don't be. Which is better: obtaining an accurate history or assuming the patient knows where their stomach pain is, when in fact it is chest pain?

Here are some examples of using reference points.

> **Example**
>
> *"If you put your hand over your tummy button, is the pain above your hand, below your hand or directly under your hand?"*
>
> Now, let's assume they have answered that it is above their hand.
>
> *"Keeping your hand over your tummy button* (they should not move from this point of reference), *is the pain closer to your hand or closer to the bone that runs between your breasts/down the centre of your chest?"*

Or

"If you drew an imaginary line around your waist, is the pain in your back above or below that line?"

If they answer that it is below that line:

"If you drew another line where the cheeks of your bottom meet your thighs, is the pain closer to the line on your waist or the one on your thighs?"

Using points of reference can really help you build a much clearer picture of where something is, and it is vital to have a good, clear understanding of where the problem is really located.

11.6.7 What has helped or made it worse?

It is important to find out if the patient has had any treatment, or remedies of any kind, that have either helped the problem or made it worse. Knowing what has already been tried prevents us from going over old ground and can also mean the treatments we could have suggested have been exhausted, so you are probably now already thinking about either prescribing medication or seeing the patient. Alternatively, we will also know what we have left in our collection of self-care measures and whether we can consider these before the need to see a patient.

Treatments will include self-medication, holistic approaches, ice/ heat packs, elevation and even positioning, for example. You need accurate and up-to-date information on what makes things better or worse.

Example: checking on medications tried

When it comes to finding out what medications have been tried, you need to be very clear on **exactly** what has been taken, rather than assuming that patients have taken the proper dose. There are five questions to ask to find out exactly what has been tried and its effect:

1. *What have they taken* (name of the medication on the bottle/ packet)?

2. *How much have they taken* (actual dosage of medication)?

3. *When did they take it and how much in total that day?*

4. *When did they take it and how much in total each day, if the symptoms have been present for more than that day?*

5. *Did it help?*

Again, never assume anything when it comes to medication. Parents will often tell you that they have given their child a 'teaspoon of paracetamol'. On probing, they will then clarify that they used a household teaspoon (which typically contains around 2–3ml and not the 5ml required for a standard dose), and that the dosage on the bottle was for a younger child (under 6 years) but the patient is 10 years old. So, the child may have been given only a quarter of the dose they could have had. Finding out exactly what has been given is crucial to your management and further advice, and yet this is often done poorly in a telephone assessment.

We also need to discover if anything has made the symptoms worsen. A patient may report that certain positions aggravate the pain, or taking a certain pain medication has made symptoms increase (for instance if they have taken ibuprofen and their stomach pain has increased; you may need to inform a patient that some medications such as anti-inflammatories are contraindicated with certain conditions such as stomach disorders).

11.7 Ascertain the history of the patient

Some of the information regarding the patient may already be available to you, or in other cases you may prefer to collect this information before going into details about the symptoms. On each call you should decide when is best to ask these questions. The key is not to be regimented in your approach and remember safety is paramount when dealing with patients over the phone. If the patient is obviously unwell, don't go into too much detail about the patient's history before dealing with what's happening at the time of the call (as we discussed in *Sections 9.3* and *9.4*).

As we have just done for history of the symptoms, we can apply a simple model or template to collect information on the patient's history. You may choose to ask these questions in any order, but some may not be relevant for each call, so you will need to judge what you require within each assessment.

Here's what the template for the history of the patient looks like:

Patient history	
Past medical history (PMH)	
Medications (including over-the-counter meds)	
Allergies	
Risk factors	

Age	
Pregnancy	
Social history	
Number of contacts	

11.7.1 What is the patient's past medical history?

Access to the patient's full medical history is now far more common with system integration, but occasionally some services aren't fully integrated and the clinician only has access to the history of contacts within their own service (typically this happens within the out-of-hours setting). This makes some clinicians nervous, but I have found that not having access to a patient's PMH encourages me to make sure I have a full understanding of the patient's history from the patient directly, rather than just reading about it. You may become a better triager when you learn not to rely on the system to tell you what has happened previously. If it is relevant to the situation that day, you should double-check the history anyway. For example, I know of a call where the clinician asked to see a patient within an hour, but the patient replied they would need more time to get to the urgent care centre because they were disabled – the clinician had no awareness of the disability because they hadn't checked the PMH thoroughly. Unfortunately, some callers are poor at relating their history or insist there is nothing of significance, before then telling you about their huge list of medications! Having access to the history can be invaluable; for example, if they have abdominal pain, have they had surgery?; if there is chest pain, is there a history of hypertension? You may need PMH information to help with your differential diagnosis, but unless it is crucial to the immediate handling of the situation, ensure the patient is safe first, before getting caught up in checking it.

11.7.2 What medications is the patient taking (including over-the-counter medications)?

Patients don't always relate taking medication to having a condition, but understanding what they are taking gives us an insight into their current health. We also need to consider whether their medications could be causing a problem or haven't been used correctly. For example, a patient may have breathing issues but they haven't been using their inhalers correctly or according to the dosage instructions. Some over-the-counter remedies are contraindicated with prescribed medications. For example, supplements that contain grapefruit may interfere with hypertension medication, or some herbal remedies such as dandelion or hibiscus can increase the effect on diuretics. We must also be vigilant about the possibility of patients trying other prescribed medication not intended for them. I have known patients to 'share' friends' medications including diuretics, pain relief (morphine) and inhalers. Elderly patients are infamous for sharing medications, so we should always check by asking *"Have you tried anything else at all for this problem? Even something that wasn't suggested by your own GP?"*.

11.7.3 Allergies

Checking on potential allergies should always be part of any assessment, especially where there is swelling of the face or breathing difficulties, or where a rash is present. If you are advising or prescribing medication, you should always make sure the patient is able to tolerate the medication and let them know how to check for any allergic reactions if they have never taken it before.

11.7.4 Are there any particular risk factors for this patient?

Any long-term conditions such as diabetes or COPD need to be considered, but be wary of associating any problem with these conditions before completing your overall assessment – you may need to discover other risk factors to help with your diagnosis. For instance, if someone has pain and swelling in their calf, sounds breathless and complains of pain in their chest, you may want to ask if they have travelled recently or been immobilised. However, sometimes focusing on these questions is more about the diagnosis than deciding if a patient needs to be seen, so be wary of spending too much time on these types of questions instead of taking action to ensure the patient is safe. The priority is to determine what care needs to be given first, and in the case of calf pain with other associated symptoms of a deep vein thrombosis (DVT) or pulmonary embolism (PE), knowing if they have travelled recently will not affect your outcome.

11.7.5 Does their age increase the risk?

Sometimes the biggest risk factor that you need to consider is simply the age of the patient. They may be too old or too young for you to take the risk of providing just telephone advice. Both patient groups can deteriorate quickly (children can also recover very quickly), but if you find that you need to see every child or every elderly patient, or have an extremely low threshold for both, consider the purpose of the triage; namely, that if a patient is going to be seen, when that should be and by whom. For example, any unwell neonate should always be seen, so your assessment is to determine when and by whom. Not all neonates are ill though (it could be a minor skin problem), so a phone call could save you and the carer an appointment. Some patients who are extremely old are still very fit individuals and their general health can be much better than someone in their 40s – once again it's about the individual, so each call should be dealt with individually.

11.7.6 Pregnancy

Any abdominal pain in women of childbearing age, or any other issue which may be related to pregnancy, is a risk and requires you to ask about their last menstrual period and whether it was normal for them. The latter question is often omitted, but a change in menstrual cycle length may be important to your working diagnosis. You need to be as sure as you can be that a pregnancy is not possible before you discount it. Sometimes questions about sexual activity, contraceptive methods and whether a woman thinks she could be pregnant or not, are redundant to a certain extent. Teenage girls may say they are not sexually active over the phone because a parent may be listening, or a woman may say they are using contraception, or their partner has had a vasectomy, but they have still become pregnant. If you are concerned that pregnancy may be an issue, it is better to treat each case individually and rule pregnancy in or out by accurate testing, rather than rely on the patient's own assessment.

11.7.7 Social history

This section has been left almost to the end of the assessment, because it could be a social issue which tips the balance between seeing a patient or not. When looking at the patient holistically, it can be the social circumstances that make it unsafe to give self-care. For example:

* For an elderly patient who lives alone you may want to arrange to visit them at home to check on their living conditions or capacity to manage.

- Where a child is not acutely unwell, but the carer doesn't seem capable of looking after the child, it may leave you wanting to arrange a face-to-face consultation to check on the carer as well as the child.

- In the case of a child who is 'at risk', i.e. they are a child who has potentially been neglected or abused, although their clinical condition at the time of the call may not sound concerning, the social circumstances may make it safer to see them physically.

If, however, the 'at risk' child is with a foster carer whom you know and trust, the child is then like every other child and not necessarily 'at risk' at the time of the call.

11.7.8 Number of contacts

The number of contacts a patient has with services can be a significant red flag, but it's not just about the number of contacts but rather:

- the number of contacts, *then*

- about what, *then*

- over how long.

A history of frequent contacts over a short period of time about the same problem sends a different signal than frequent contacts about differing things over a short period of time. If a caller keeps ringing back about the same problem over a short period of time, something isn't right. Either they have not been reassured or educated enough, or the clinician may be missing something. If a caller rings several times in a short period of time but each time it's to report something completely different, there is less of a clinical risk and perhaps more of a dependency situation. Then again, several contacts about lots of different things over several months doesn't necessarily indicate any risk. Also, if you have a patient who hasn't been seen in surgery for several years, they may be a higher risk than a 'frequent flyer', because they rarely seek care and by doing so, a significant issue is often indicated.

Unfortunately, there have been several cases where the number of contacts has been a huge red flag, but not recognised as such. The death of a patient called Penny Campbell in 2005 following eight contacts to an out-of-hours service, of which only the first and last resulted in a face-to-face assessment, was the catalyst for significant changes to the recording and sharing of information. Some clinicians will ensure a patient is seen if there is contact more than twice about the same problem, but there is still some value in carrying out another telephone assessment to ensure safety regarding when and by whom they are seen.

Take-home message

When taking a history there are several aspects to consider initially to establish the patient's immediate condition. A key component before going into detail, however, is to find out the caller's agenda, because it will help you manage their expectations. Once you can progress with the assessment, develop a structured approach to find out about the history of the symptoms as well as the history of the patient.

Chapter 12
Stage 3 of taking a call: the management plan

> **Key points**
> - Provide one last opportunity to discuss any concerns before offering your advice/outcome
> - Try to avoid getting 'hijacked'
> - Provide any self-care advice clearly and ensure the caller's understanding of it
> - Make sure everyone is clear on what to do next and document this accordingly

12.1 One last question

You are now at the point where you can offer your advice, but you might want to check you haven't missed anything. However, be careful of simply asking *"Was there anything else you feel you wanted to discuss or ask me about?"*. By asking this question in this way, there is the possibility of getting 'hijacked'. This is a term I like to use when you are just about to end a call but then someone says, *"Whilst I have you….."* or *"Could I also just ask you about….."* and you end up discussing something else entirely and the caller 'hijacks' your time and the call.

If you've clarified the reason for the call at the beginning and asked the caller what they hope you will be able to do for them (see *Section 11.4* for 'what's their agenda?'), you shouldn't get 'hijacked' too often. If you suspect someone is likely to ask about something else at the end of the call as they've done it before, make sure you ask them again at the beginning of the call what they wish to talk to you about and perhaps say:

> *"So, just to be clear, we are going to talk about* (state the problem they rang about). *Was there anything else at all you wanted to discuss or ask me about?"*.

If they still surprise you at the end of the call or 'hijack' you, you can decide if it's appropriate to continue to talk about another issue or remind them that you asked them what they needed to discuss at the beginning and they failed to mention a second issue then. You can then suggest that they can either place another call or discuss the second issue when you see them if they are coming in. This is called 'controlling the call' whereby you aren't being led in a different direction or manipulated into a second assessment when it's not appropriate.

A better approach is to phrase the question *"Was there anything else **about this problem today** that you feel we haven't discussed?"* before you begin your management plan. Sometimes, there is a hidden agenda which may only be discovered by allowing the caller this final opportunity to disclose their concerns.

This question also directly links to the initial probing question of *"What were you hoping I'd be able to do for you today?"*. If you have established their agenda at the beginning of the call, you shouldn't really need to check again at the end if there is anything else that's worrying them, but it reassures you and the caller that you've addressed their concerns.

Before you offer your outcome or advice, it's important to check that your understanding of the problem still matches that of the caller by summarising the conversation as you comprehend it. You may also need to take a moment to reflect on what's been said, so give yourself some thinking time to decide if you have everything you need for your decision-making. The examples below show a couple of useful phrases to give yourself a bit of thinking time.

Example

"I just want to pull our conversation together to make sure we have everything we need before we decide what to do. I'm going to go quiet for a few seconds whilst I go through it all in my head."

Or perhaps more simply:

"Just give me a second while I think through everything."

If you have kept to the structure suggested in *Chapter 11*, you should find it much easier to decide that you have completed your assessment and can confidently offer your advice.

12.2 Giving self-care advice

Part of most assessments will be providing information on how the caller or patient can manage their symptoms themselves – known as self-care advice. However, sometimes the clinician offers too much material by way of self-care advice. For some conditions, like influenza for instance, there can be large amounts of information that could be useful. This can make the call exceptionally long, both verbally and in the subsequent documenting of the call (it should all be documented). So, even though this could all be excellent evidence-based advice, it is important to be wary of providing too much self-care material.

One way to make sure you give focused self-care information, whilst keeping the attention of the caller, is to consider giving only three or four pieces of key information; stick to what is necessary from a clinical risk point of view.

If you feel the patient needs more than just three or four bits of self-care advice, then make sure you break it down into a numbered list which will help the caller with their ability to recall everything.

12.3 Be clear on what happens next

Once you have reached an outcome, it's essential that you and your caller are clear on what the next steps are. I have had many callers who have accepted 'self-care' and, after spending a couple of minutes talking through what they should do to manage their symptoms themselves, they have then asked, *"That's great but when do I see the doctor?"*. Obviously I wasn't as clear as I thought in explaining my outcome!

To avoid this happening, you may want to say:

> *"Just to make sure we both understand what's going to happen next, would you mind telling me what we agreed you will do? I want to make sure I was clear in the way I explained it".*

Remember the earlier section on communication and getting the caller to repeat back their understanding (see *Section 5.3*)? The same technique is useful here for both giving self-care advice and checking the patient understands what's going to happen next. Once you and the caller are clear on the next steps, it is equally important that you record this in their notes as well.

Take-home message

Check that your final understanding of the problem matches that of the caller and after offering your advice, make sure everyone involved is clear on the next steps and how to carry out self-care advice.

Chapter 13
Safety-netting

Safety-netting is the term generally used to identify what the caller/patient needs to look for that would indicate a worsening situation; the sections below describe in detail what's needed for good safety-netting. Safety-netting at the end of a call is probably one of the most important parts of the call, especially when you decide not to see the patient face-to-face. Always remember, **the *provision* of safety-netting advice is about protecting the patient, whilst the *documentation* of the advice given is about protecting the clinician**.

Most clinicians close a call that's resulted in self-care with what is termed a 'general worsening statement' such as, *"Ring back if you are worried about anything at all"*. This is one of the weakest forms of safety-netting, because it's too general and non-specific. It doesn't provide information on what to look out for specifically, and simply gives permission for the caller to ring back if they are worried about anything.

You also risk getting calls in which the 'concern' is that they are continuing to experience the same symptoms, even if this is exactly what you would expect given the short time that has elapsed. Alternatively, and more worryingly, the patient may not recognise that something has changed or worsened enough to warrant a call because you hadn't gone into detail about what to look out for; so, they don't call anyone and harm could occur subsequently.

Even if you are arranging a face-to-face consultation (including an urgent response such as a home visit within 1 hour or advising the patient that they go to A&E), you should consider adding in some safety-netting advice about what to do if things change or worsen before the patient is seen or before medical assistance arrives.

13.1   What do they need to look out for?

You need to give information to the patient on what *specific* signs and symptoms to look out for that would indicate a worsening condition; if possible, confine this to only three or four things. Any more than that, and the caller is likely to forget what you said. It also helps the clinician to focus on what's really important. You could also ask the caller to write down your instructions and read them back to you to ensure clarity and understanding on both sides. If you want to cover more than three or four things, consider giving them in another format, such as emailing or texting the caller a link to a website with more details, or by sending a leaflet out.

13.2   When should the caller seek help again?

You will need to provide a clear time frame in which to look out for changing or worsening symptoms. Be careful of non-specific time frames such as *"this may go on for 3–5 days"* because the caller may be confused about whether to seek further advice on day 3, day 4, day 5, or even wait until day 6. See the example below for how this might be done:

Clinician: *"With this kind of viral infection, children typically begin to feel better by day 3 (which will be tomorrow), but they can be poorly for up to 5 days. I'd like you to keep an eye on things, but if there is no improvement at all by day 5 (which will be Thursday morning), you must call the surgery and let us know so we can have another chat about things. However, if any symptoms seem to get worse at any time, please call us back immediately and don't wait until Thursday."*

In some cases such as back pain, the pain can be there for several weeks, but you don't want the patient to keep ringing back to tell you that they are still experiencing pain, which is what you would have expected. Similarly, you don't want them waiting to contact you if things aren't improving in the way they should, so the advice on when to call back will be more complicated (see below):

Clinician: *"With this kind of back pain, I'm afraid it's not unusual to experience some discomfort for up to 6 weeks, but I'm going to tell you how I would expect things to be during that time. You may have significant pain for the first 2 weeks, but it should be helped by using the medication and other treatments we've discussed. As long as things improve a little each day, you will be OK to manage things yourself. However, if the pain gets worse despite the treatments, or any new symptoms appear (as we've just discussed), you must let someone know immediately (we'll discuss who that should be next). After 6 weeks, if there are any symptoms or discomfort that's still present or that worries you, call the surgery and we can have another chat about it."*

You can see that by giving the patient an accurate picture of what to expect and when, you should avoid unnecessary contacts whilst ensuring the patient knows what to expect and when they need to seek further help.

13.3 Who should the caller contact if they do need further advice?

You also need to be clear on which service the patient should contact for additional help if their symptoms change or worsen. Consider whether this should be a second contact with your service or another service. For example:

- If the original call was taken at a GP surgery but things change overnight, should the caller contact the out-of-hours service or wait until the surgery is open again?

- If it's the weekend, they would need to contact the out-of-hours service, but is the patient clear about how to do that? You don't want a deteriorating patient to delay contacting someone simply because they are unsure of what to do if the surgery is closed.

- If the call was originally taken out-of-hours, you should advise the caller on whether to contact their own surgery when it opens or to ring the out-of-hours service if it's still open.

- In extreme cases, you may have to advise that the caller phone 999 or attend A&E rather than waste time contacting a primary care service if the patient has significantly deteriorated.

In the following example, you can see how these elements would look in a real call:

You have assessed a child with symptoms suggestive of non-complex viral infection. The following script is an example of what the safety-netting that you'll give to the parent in this case may look like:

Clinician: *"I'm going to give you some information on **what to look out for** over the next 3 days.*

Firstly, make sure they are responding normally and you can wake them up if you need to.

Secondly, keep an eye on how much and how often they vomit. I'd expect the vomiting to be reducing in amount and frequency, not getting worse.

Thirdly, keep monitoring their temperature. It might not come down to normal, but it should respond to the medication, even just a little bit.

Finally, look out for any new symptoms or see if anything gets worse.

*I'm going to ask you shortly to repeat everything back to me to make sure I've been clear, but these symptoms may go on for another couple of days. If any symptoms are still present on Friday, which is day 5 since it all started, I need to know about it. This is **when** you need to call me back if nothing changes.*

*However, if any symptoms get worse or you are concerned in any way, either call the surgery or, if we are closed, you should call the out-of-hours service **(who)**. I wouldn't expect this to happen at all, but if they suddenly seem to be delirious or unresponsive, don't be frightened to dial 999.*

Would you mind repeating back to me the information that I've just given you, to make sure that you are happy with what to look out for, when to contact someone and who to contact?"

> **Take-home message**
>
> To truly protect your patient, you need to provide clear details on what to look out for, when to contact someone again and who to contact. This make take a little bit of time but in order to ensure the safety of the patient, especially if you aren't arranging a face-to-face consult, you have to be specific and comprehensive in your advice.

Chapter 14
How to close a call

> **Key points**
>
> - There are two elements to closing a call – the clinical closure and knowing how to say goodbye
> - Develop phrases for saying goodbye

Closing a call can be one of the hardest parts of triage and one that many clinicians struggle with. There are two parts to the closing of the call: reaching the end of the consultation clinically, where you feel there is nothing else you can do for the patient, then actually saying goodbye and disconnecting (which is not always easy to do).

14.1 Clinical closure

Clinical closure is when you reach your decision about the outcome and indicate this to the caller because there isn't anything else you need to know or discuss. We discussed in *Section 12.1* the need for taking a bit of time to think everything through, so this will help you in confirming that there aren't any other questions you need to ask before reaching your conclusion. You need to be confident that your outcome is the right one from a safety point of view. We will address the issue of non-compliance in *Chapter 15* but, once you have reached your decision, I would strongly advise against backtracking or changing your mind because this will create a lack of trust from the caller and will leave you feeling less confident – remember confidence is vital in telephone assessments.

14.2 How to say goodbye

One of the trickiest parts of a phone consultation can actually be ending the call without making the caller feel alienated, or disgruntled at the fact that you are ending a call when they may be happy to keep chatting to you! Over the phone, it is more difficult to imply that the interaction must now end. If you were face-to-face in the surgery, you would begin to conclude the consultation by perhaps closing the notes down, handing over a prescription, rising from your chair and walking to the door, or even walking out of the office with the patient to suggest the consultation is over. We can't use these approaches over the phone, so you need to consider developing your own 'scripts' or phrases for bringing the call to an end and saying goodbye. Some phrases I like to use are shown below:

Example

"Well, I hope you are feeling better soon. Hopefully we won't need to talk again but you know to ring back if you feel you need to. Goodbye."

or

"I am sure things will get better soon but if not, remember everything we discussed about what to try and when to contact someone if things change or worsen. Bye now."

or

"We will see you in the surgery (names time/day) *but please forgive me, I have to go as I'm needed to help another patient, so I'll say goodbye now. Bye."*

The gold standard within commercial telephone services is that the caller should disconnect first, but in the clinical world this can lead to a conversation that goes on and on. If you know you have covered everything and everyone is clear on the next steps (see *Section 12.3*), simply say goodbye and put the phone down.

Take-home message

Once you have reached your conclusion and you know there is nothing else you can offer, be prepared to close the call with phrases that don't alienate the caller.

Chapter 15
What to do if patients don't agree with your advice

Key points

- Not all callers will accept your advice; there are times when that's OK, but also times when patient safety concerns mean that you may need to go against their wishes
- Ensure that the caller is making an informed decision about what they plan to do
- Consider the safety of a child or a vulnerable adult if the carer doesn't want to comply with your decision

Despite your best efforts to offer the safest and most appropriate outcome for your patient, there will be times when this advice isn't accepted, or you can't reach a mutually agreed outcome. So, what should you do if this happens?

It's always best to anticipate a potential conflict and have a 'Plan B' ready that still ensures that the patient is as safe as they can be, given their age and the nature of the call. However, at times we need to accept that patients have the right to disregard our advice. We have talked about patient demand versus expectation in *Section 2.3* but sometimes we just can't offer what the patient wants, for example:

- a specific appointment time/day

- when their agenda isn't appropriate, such as a request for a home visit which is unreasonable given the nature of the complaint and the patient's ability to attend a clinic or surgery

- a request for inappropriate medication which would be unsafe.

Sometimes, we must accept that what the caller or patient chooses to do is exactly that, i.e. their choice. But there are times when that wouldn't be appropriate, such as when the patient is a child or a vulnerable adult.

15.1 What to do when the patient is a child or a vulnerable adult

If the patient is a child and therefore unable to decide what they want to do, or an adult who is considered vulnerable due to capacity issues, you must stress to the carer the importance of why they should follow your advice, but also clearly state the reasons for your outcome/diagnosis. **You need to ensure that they are making an informed decision** (see example below) and then hopefully they will acquiesce to your advice.

Example

You have assessed a child and your diagnosis is that they have a significant upper respiratory tract infection which needs further examination, but the parent is reluctant to bring them into the surgery because the weather is poor. It's not that they can't get to the surgery, they just prefer not to. A good way of handling this is to say:

*"**From what you have told me**, the reason I am suggesting (name the child) is seen in the surgery within (state the time frame), is because **I can't rule out** a chest infection. I really need to see them to make sure they don't require antibiotics, or any other treatment. If they don't get the right treatment, this could turn into a more significant infection like pneumonia and they could become very poorly indeed."*

The key phrases here are "**from what you've told me**" and "**I can't rule out**", which clearly states what the problem is likely to be (your initial diagnosis). Both phrases tell the carer that your advice is based on what they have told you, combined with your judgement of what might occur if they don't bring the child in to be seen. Most carers will respond to this, but if you are still struggling to achieve compliance, remember that your concerns and duty of care are to the child.

If you have advised that a child should be seen within two hours, but the carer can't get to the surgery for at least four hours due to transport issues for instance, be very careful about moving the goal posts. If you have made a clinical judgement that the child needs further care and assessment within a certain time frame and the child can't get to you, your 'Plan B' may be that you will have to visit the child. In a busy practice, this isn't always possible because you have other patients and other duties to take care of. In this case, 'Plan C' may be to suggest another facility closer to them, such as an Urgent Care Centre. Failing that, and depending on the severity of the illness, you may even want to consider transportation to hospital, but this is extreme and shouldn't be necessary if primary care is what's required. The example below demonstrates how this conversation may happen after the initial 'Plan A' has been given in the previous example:

Clinician: *"If you are sure you can't get to the surgery in the next couple of hours* (Plan A), *let's see what else we can do"*

Carer: *"Could you come and see them at home Doctor?"*

Clinician: *"I'm afraid I can't leave the surgery to come and see* (names the child) *at home, as I'm needed here to see other patients. Also, we have very strict guidelines on when home visits should be done and I'm sorry but this wouldn't meet the criteria, as they should be seen in surgery (Plan B)"*

Carer: *"Oh well, what else can I do? I just couldn't get into the surgery for about 4 hours as my partner has the car and I couldn't manage the two little ones by myself on the bus"*

Clinician: *"Is there somewhere else closer to you that you could go along to? I think there is an Urgent Care Centre or Walk-in Centre not far from you. Could you go there in the next 2 hours* (Plan C)?"*

Carer: *"Yes, I can walk there with the pushchair"*

Clinician: *"That's great. I can ring them and tell them you'll be going along in the next 2 hours so you shouldn't have to wait long."*

Many clinicians believe that if they are clear on what to do if symptoms worsen, then surely, it's the carer's responsibility to bring the child in when they can. This seems reasonable, but if some harm came to the child outside the time frame in which you asked to see them, you may be held accountable despite telling the carer what to look out for or be concerned about in the meantime. Your duty of care is to the child first and foremost. Denying the child access to healthcare, i.e. if the carer has the ability to bring the child to the surgery and travelling will not cause the child to deteriorate, could arguably be reported as a safeguarding matter.

The overall consideration should always be what's best for the child. As much as a carer may be abusing the service and demanding an inappropriate outcome, if you are worried about the wellbeing of a child, your decision should always be to ensure their safety first. You may wish to seek further advice on the handling of this situation from local leads or the organisation in which you work.

15.2 What if the patient is an adult?

When it comes to adults, your approach is likely to be different. If you are sure that they need a face-to-face assessment and you give the patient a time frame for attendance, and the travelling will not cause them to decline, then it's a different set of care rules. The competent adult patient can make a decision about their own care themselves and that may not be what you suggest. However, it is always better to try to gain compliance.

Once again, you should **make sure they are making an informed decision**. State very clearly why they need to be seen (or not, as the case may be), i.e. your diagnosis, or be honest and tell them they need further assessment to reach an accurate diagnosis. A patient can refuse your advice, but your duty of care means they need to fully understand why you have reached your decision and diagnosis, if possible.

One way to gain the patient's cooperation (especially when they won't accept a higher level of care) is what nurses often refer to as a 'duty to terrify'! Personally, I have used this kind of approach several times with elderly patients who have refused an ambulance when they have described symptoms suggestive of a cardiac event (see the example below).

Example

"From what you told me was happening, you could be having a heart attack. Are you sure I can't arrange an ambulance for you?"

If they still decline, I will then say:

"As I said, from what you've told me, I can't rule out the possibility of a heart attack. If you don't let me arrange an ambulance straight away, you may die."

At this point they usually agree, but if they don't and there is no reason to suspect any mental capacity issues, I will finish by saying:

"OK, I will make a note of the fact that I have strongly advised an ambulance as I suspect a possible heart attack, and you have declined it".

Make it clear to the caller/patient that you are documenting their decision not to accept your outcome ('declining' is a less confrontational way of saying it than 'refused'), but it is their right to do so. At this point, I usually find that they will accept my recommendation, fortunately.

Ultimately, if the patient is an adult with no capacity issues, they can refuse your advice.

Take-home message

Although we should always strive for joint decision-making, it's not always possible. If the patient is making an informed decision, we must allow them to do so. In the case of a child or vulnerable adult you should aim to have an alternative plan, but if the carer won't comply, remember that your duty of care is to the vulnerable patient, so you may have to consider your safeguarding protocols to ensure the patient is seen.

Chapter 16
Documentation and record-keeping

Key points

- Record-keeping can be in the form of electronic notes or a voice recording
- Documentation of telephone calls is very similar to face-to-face encounters, but there are a few exceptions
- Develop your own structure for your documentation
- Wherever possible, voice record your calls

Telephone triage may have two forms of documentation or what is considered record-keeping – the electronic record of the patient and a voice recording of the call (digital). Some services still don't voice record, however, so you should never assume that a voice recording will exist. Voice recordings are an accepted form of record-keeping as far as the General Medical Council (GMC) and the Nursing and Midwifery Council (NMC) are concerned and they are admissible in court. We will talk more about voice recording in *Section 16.4* but, as with any form of digital information, a voice recording can be corrupted or of poor quality, or can even be lost, so your primary record should always be considered as the electronic notes. Ensure that any information that is relevant is recorded in the notes and try to avoid using the voice recording as your primary record, or omit documenting relevant information in the notes because you consider it to be 'on the tape', for the reasons just stated.

Clear documentation is necessary to relay what's happening to the patient and for future contacts so that everyone is clear on what's occurred and what may be needed next. Your documentation is also a key component in protecting you from legal liability and needs to be sufficient to support your decision-making and, if necessary, to defend your actions if called into question.

I've witnessed a huge variation amongst colleagues when it comes to documentation, especially when there's no Clinical Decision Support System (CDSS) providing the structure. I've even seen people use 'to be seen' or 'appointment given' as the only documentation, with no other entry at all as a record of the interaction, other than a date and time stamp! I've also seen some very expansive notes where clinicians have documented absolutely everything that has been discussed, usually to try to protect themselves from legal accountability if they chose not to see the patient.

So how does documentation of a telephone assessment differ from that for a face-to-face encounter? In my opinion, very little. When you see a patient in surgery, you will document the salient points, your diagnosis and any treatments you advised or referrals you made. You won't necessarily write out the whole of the conversation that took place. You will also record any clinical findings you established. Essentially, the same principles apply to a telephone encounter: documentation of the salient points, your diagnosis, treatments recommended, referrals made and any clinical findings that you either asked about or got the caller to carry out on your behalf.

In the same way as I've recommended a call structure and a structure for taking a history, you should develop a structure for your documentation. The template for taking a history suggested in *Chapter 11* can also be used for documentation purposes. Your record should show clearly what was happening and why you made the decision that you did, but without being so long that it's adding to your workload or affecting your efficiency.

We know that from a medicolegal point of view, "*if it's not written down, it didn't happen*" is the accepted norm. This isn't true literally, because it could be on the voice recording, but even without the recording it doesn't mean you *didn't* discuss something. However, governing bodies will typically side with the caller if there is a dispute between what you say happened and the caller's recollection in the absence of evidence to the contrary, either on a voice recording or in the notes.

The following sections are some suggestions for additional information you might consider recording.

16.1 Who told you what?

If at any time you spoke to a third party who contributed information that was either not also given to you by the patient, or was different to the patient's declarations, make sure you make it clear in the notes who told you what. Ideally, obtain the third party's full name, or at least their relationship with the patient, and record this as well.

16.2 Specific safety-netting advice

This is a crucial part of your documentation and the full safety-netting advice you gave should be documented in case the caller denies the instructions given for contacting you again, or chooses not to follow your advice about going to A&E, for instance. We discussed safety-netting in detail in *Chapter 13*, but your documentation of this needs to be equally robust. In the same way that safety-netting can easily be too vague, e.g. *"call back if you're worried"*, so too can the documentation, e.g. "safety-netting given" or "red flags discussed". Notes like this don't provide the detail that may be needed to protect you in the absence of a voice recording if some harm later befalls the patient. I would recommend that you provide details on what you advised to look out for, when to contact someone if anything changes or worsens, and who to contact (see the example below).

> **Example**
>
> This could be your documentation for the safety-netting given to a parent whose child has been vomiting, with a mild temperature and who has accepted self-care:
>
> *"Advised to observe for reduced responsiveness, increase in temperature above 38°C for more than 24 hours, weakness, abdominal pain or reduction in input of fluids. To call back if any of these symptoms occur, or to ring 999 if patient shows lack of responsiveness or starts vomiting blood or dark emesis".*

If something goes wrong following a triage that wasn't voice recorded, the safety-netting and more specifically what was discussed with regard to what to look out for, can be one of the biggest points of contention – the caller may deny being told what to look out for or what to do if things worsened. Remember **the provision of the safety-netting advice is to protect the patient, but the documentation is to protect ourselves**.

16.3 What the caller plans to do

Document what the caller or patient plans to do exactly – whether they agreed to your recommended advice or not. The caller may deny what was advised or offered, or simply not turn up to an appointment you gave them, for example. If the caller disagrees with you at all, document what they said they were going to do. Also, for the purposes of ensuring anyone else involved in the patient's care understands your decision-making, it's important that you have documented your advice and the caller's choice. For instance, if you have tried to offer self-care management but the caller insists on seeing someone, document clearly what you advised and why, so any other clinicians involved will understand why the patient has received an appointment when it may not have been clinically appropriate.

16.4 Should you voice record your calls?

Out-of-hours services now always voice record their calls, but some organisations still don't use voice recording equipment. I think that all telephone services should record their calls – there are far more advantages than disadvantages to voice recording and these advantages are listed below.

- The biggest advantage is that they are an additional record of what happened and can often provide more information than was recorded in the notes – most importantly how the patient or caller sounded. In *Section 5.4.2* we discussed how 84% of a telephone interaction is down to interpretation of the tone of voice; a clinical record or document doesn't show this unless the clinician chooses to write down their impression of how the caller or patient sounded. A written document is also only the clinician's version of things. A voice recording may support the clinician further, although it may of course contradict them.

- Voice recordings are an invaluable tool when it comes to your own education and improvement. Nothing is as powerful as hearing your own calls when it comes to learning and development. You will hear what you do well, what works as far as phraseology goes, but also what is unsuccessful, or what you may need to change – such as interrupting callers, talking over the top of them or having long silences during your call.

- Knowing you are voice recorded can help you moderate your behaviour and have a similar effect on your caller.

- Clinical audit or quality assurance is far more valuable when based on voice recordings, because it's fairer to the clinician. It provides full details of the call, including how the patient sounded, and so can indicate where some of the clinician's observations may have come from, compared to a documented conversation. Statistical analysis doesn't show the quality of the call.

- I think the most important reason for voice recording is that it provides authentic and unquestionable evidence of what happened, if there is an untoward incident or a complaint. It can save hours or even days of time when it comes to investigations, which in turn can save thousands of pounds. If harm has come to a patient, you know exactly what was discussed and removes the issue of whether or not something was said, if there is a discrepancy in recollections. During my work as an expert witness, the voice recording is priceless and instrumental in my ability to comment on what happened. I wouldn't accept instructions on a case unless a voice recording was available, because the patient's documented notes only reflect the clinician's account, which unfortunately may not always be accurate. Conversely, many complaints aren't upheld after listening to the voice recording, because the caller often misheard what was said or their recollection of what they thought they had said was wrong.

Take-home message

Your documentation is about making sure everyone is clear on what was discussed for future care, but it's also about protecting yourself and making sure it's clear to everyone why you did what you did. Voice recordings are an invaluable tool when it comes to record-keeping.

Chapter 17
The role of the GP receptionist

> ### Key points
>
> - Receptionists are usually the first point of contact for patients and therefore need the right skills
> - The role of the receptionist directly impacts the quality and quantity of the call backs the clinician must make
> - Receptionists are becoming 'care navigators'
> - The work of the receptionist can help streamline the patient journey and reduce the workload of the clinician

In surgeries, calls are initially handled by a non-clinician, usually the GP receptionists, before they appear on the call-back list for the clinician. The role of the receptionist nowadays (and post-pandemic in particular) is a complex and difficult one. Having trained and observed hundreds of receptionists over the years, I have a newfound respect and admiration for the work they do and a greater understanding of how their work directly impacts that of the clinician. The roles of the receptionist and the clinical triager are interlinked and it would be inappropriate to underestimate the responsibility of the person who first takes the call.

Under the pressures of today's primary care services, surgeries have begun to recognise that receptionists are much more involved in managing the workload of the clinical team and the role has developed to that of 'care navigators'. These staff are expected to carry out a form of 'triage' to identify the callers' needs and filter out those calls that don't need to go anywhere near a clinician. A few internal studies that I've seen in practices have shown that 20–33% of calls that come into the practice could be managed by receptionists or other administrative staff and don't need to be passed to a clinician to deal with. In other cases, a patient may have asked for a GP appointment, but a nurse or pharmacist may have been able to help and so the receptionist has successfully diverted that call and reduced the number of appointments for the GP. Patients may also try to make an appointment with a GP practice when they should be going to another healthcare resource such as A&E or a Minor Injury Unit.

To be able to direct the patient to the correct person, the receptionist must find out the reason for the call or request for an appointment. Prior to the pandemic, many surgeries would only ask the reason for the contact if the patient asked for an urgent or same-day appointment, or an appointment with the nurse. As discussed in *Chapter 1*, during the pandemic, surgeries were operating a 'total triage' system, whereby patients would be assessed over the phone before being giving a face-to-face appointment. This total triage system required receptionists to ascertain the reason for the contact. Many surgeries have chosen to retain this system post-pandemic and receptionists are now much more comfortable and confident in asking patients the reason for the appointment request. Unfortunately, however, asking what the problem is requires a particular skill set to gain sufficient information without conducting a full clinical assessment, and many receptionists receive little or no training in these skills.

Having observed receptionists at close quarters, I am pleased to report there are very few of the notorious 'dragons' left! Those autocratic, unfriendly, nosy gatekeepers who saw it as their job to prevent any but the most ill patients from seeing the GP have mainly gone. Most receptionists are doing a difficult job to the best of their ability, and yet they are subjected to the most abusive language and behaviour from all directions. General practice would crumble without skilled receptionists and their role is vital within a telephone triage system. Their ability to signpost to the right provider and prioritise the urgency of call backs or face-to-face appointments is crucial to patient safety and managing the workload of the clinicians.

The receptionists can also assist the clinician with some of the considerations necessary when dealing with phone calls, such as:

- consent for the clinician to identify themselves or not, to whoever answers the phone

- whether or not to leave voicemail messages

- ensuring the correct demographics (in particular contact numbers) have been entered

- confidentiality and consent issues.

The assistance of a good reception team is an invaluable one when it comes to getting appropriate calls onto your call-back list and in streamlining access to the patient. Do consider good quality training to ensure your receptionist staff have the best knowledge and skills to handle those initial calls – it will pay dividends when it comes to your own workload!

Take-home message

The role of the receptionist is key to the smooth running of your systems and in managing patient safety at the first point of contact. Using the skills of the receptionist appropriately will help with the workload of the clinician and will help ensure patients get the right care, by the right person and at the right time.

Chapter 18
Summary

Throughout this book I hope I have convinced you of the value of assessing patients over the telephone (whether you call it a telephone triage or telephone consultation), but I am cognisant of the inherent risks of assessing patients without physically examining them or simply 'eyeballing' your patient. Having an awareness of the risks will help you determine if the risk is such that you need to arrange for your patient to be seen, or if you can confidently manage their care over the phone.

Outlined below are some of the key points you should consider when carrying out a telephone assessment:

1. Don't prejudge the outcome or the nature of the call.

2. Things that influence your decision-making include operational capacity, who is going to see the patient, your own experiences and personality traits, and the patient's demands.

3. The primary aim of a phone assessment should be to decide whether a patient needs to be seen. Although you should aim for a diagnosis, if the patient is going to be seen (because they demand it or you are concerned about them) the diagnosis can be confirmed then, so don't waste time trying to ensure you have the correct diagnosis on the phone if it's not going to change your outcome of a face-to-face appointment.

4. If the caller trusts you, they are more likely to give you better information and accept your advice, so always strive to engage with your caller.

5. Be aware of some of the most common risks (including confirmation bias and third party callers) that you may encounter, then decide on a call-by-call basis how you want to manage those risks.

6. Be careful of making any assumptions – clarify as much as possible.

7. Time constraints can rush you to premature conclusions and can affect your tone of voice, so try not to hurry through a call.

8. Ensure you communicate effectively by having an equal amount of listening and talking throughout the call, otherwise there's a higher chance of miscommunication.

9. Tone of voice can account for 84% of the interaction – yours and the caller's – so be aware of how you sound and what you are interpreting from their tone of voice and not just the words being used.

10. Most calls may require a mixture of questioning techniques, but facilitative questions are better than closed questions when possible.

11. Avoid multiple questions or asking the same question several times.

12. You can teach yourself to help callers self-examine, but don't attempt this if there is any doubt about your ability to communicate effectively with the caller.

13. Never take symptoms out of context of the patient's overall condition.

14. Make the right preparations for taking a call, including smiling as you introduce yourself.

15. Be careful of how and when you introduce yourself if you don't know the patient or their social situation.

16. Establish the caller's agenda as soon as possible.

17. Develop your own structure for taking a history so that you cover the relevant points and streamline your approach to be as time-efficient as possible.

18. The provision of safety-netting advice is about protecting the patient; the documentation is about protecting the clinician.

19. Callers may not always agree with our recommendations but know when it's safe to allow them to decide their own care or when to override their wishes for their own safety.

20. Your documentation should include your impression of how the patient sounded and support your decision-making, but voice record calls whenever possible.

Wherever you are carrying out telephone assessments, I would urge you to seek out formal training if you have not already done so. Since the pandemic, many companies are now offering training in this clinical skill but, as with all things, the quality of this training is hugely variable, so seek out a company that has a good reputation. My own company, Telelearning, offers classroom-based and virtual training for clinical and non-clinical staff (see www.telelearning.co.uk for details). The Royal College of General Practitioners (RCGP) has offered training on telephone triage and consultation skills for over a decade, and continues to do so.

However you approach it, I wish you the best of luck in your future telephone work!